Birdshot Retinochoroidopathy: Volume 2

Edited by

C. Stephen Foster, MD, FACS, FACR

Birdshot Retinochoroidopathy: Volume 2

ISBN: 978-0-9994905-4-9

(Also available in eBook format)

Ocular Immunology and Uveitis Foundation

1440 Main Street, Suite 201

Waltham, MA 02451

www.uveitis.org

Contributors

Bharti Arya, MRCOphth
Medical Retina and Uveitis Service
Moorfields Eye Hospital
London, UK

Bahram Bodaghi, MD, PhD, FEBO
DHU Vision and Handicaps
Department of Ophthalmology
Hôpital Pitié-Salpêtrière
Paris, France

Antoine P. Brézin, MD, PhD
Université Paris Descartes
Hôpital Cochin, Service d'Ophtalmologie
Assistance Publique Hôpitaux de Paris
Paris, France

C. Stephen Foster, MD, FACS, FACR
Founder and President
Massachusetts Eye Research and Surgery Institution
Clinical Professor
Harvard Medical School
Boston, MA, USA

Carl P. Herbort Jr., MD, PhD
University of Lausanne
Retinal and Inflammatory Eye Disease
Centre for Ophthalmic Specialized Care (COS)
Clinic Montchoisi
Lausanne, Switzerland

Henry J. Kaplan, MD, FACS
Department of Ophthalmology & Visual Sciences
Kentucky Lions Eye Center
University of Louisville
Louisville, KY, USA

Phuc LeHoang, MD, PhD
Professor of Ophthalmology
DHU Vision and Handicaps
Inflammation-Immunopathology-Biotherapy Department
Université Pierre et Marie Curie
Hôpital Pitié-Salpêtrière
Paris, France

Ralph D. Levinson, MD
Professor of Health Sciences
Cornea and Uveitis Division, Jules Stein Eye Institute David Geffen School of Medicine at the University of California, Los Angeles
Los Angeles, CA, USA

Breno R. Lima, MD
Laboratory of Immunology
National Eye Institute, National Institutes of Health
Bethesda, MD, USA

Robert B. Nussenblatt, MD, MPH
Laboratory of Immunology
National Eye Institute, National Institutes of Health
Bethesda, MD, USA

Marina Papadia
Retinal and Inflammatory Eye Disease
Centre for Ophthalmic Specialized Care (COS)
Clinic Montchoisi
Lausanne, Switzerland
Ospedale Antero Micone
Genova, Italy

Carlos Pavesio, MD, FRCOphth
Consultant Ophthalmologist
Moorfields Eye Hospital
London, UK

Niloofar Piri, MD
Department of Ophthalmology & Visual Sciences
Kentucky Lions Eye Center
University of Louisville
Louisville, KY, USA

H. Nida Sen, MD, MHS
Laboratory of Immunology
National Eye Institute, National Institutes of Health
Bethesda, MD, USA

Albert T. Vitale, MD
Clinical Professor, Director of Uveitis Division
Dept. of Ophthalmology and Visual Sciences
John A. Moran Eye Center
Salt Lake City, UT, USA

To all patients with birdshot retinochoroidopathy

Contents

Chapter 1
Definition and Etiology
Antoine P. Brézin

Chapter 2
Epidemiology and Natural History
Albert T. Vitale

Chapter 3
Evidence of Autoimmunity
Breno R. Lima, H. Nida Sen, Robert B. Nussenblatt

Chapter 4
Immunogenetics
Ralph D. Levinson

Chapter 5
Outcomes with Corticosteroids
Carlos Pavesio, Bharti Arya

Chapter 6
Outcomes with Immunomodulatory Therapy
C. Stephen Foster

Chapter 7
Best Monitoring Practices
Henry J. Kaplan, Niloofar Piri

Chapter 8
Rectifications in the Appraisal of BSRC
Carl P. Herbort Jr., Marina Papadia

Chapter 9
Determinants of Remission and Cure
Phuc LeHoang

Chapter 10
Biologic Response Modifier Therapy
Antoine P. Brézin

Chapter 11
Corticosteroid Implant Therapy
Henry J. Kaplan, Niloofar Piri

Chapter 12
New Therapeutic Strategies in Development
Bahram Bodaghi

Chapter 13
Identifying Gaps in Knowledge
Albert T. Vitale

Chapter 14
Bridging the Gaps in Knowledge
Robert B. Nussenblatt

Preface

Birdshot retinochoroidopathy (BSRC) is a progressively blinding autoimmune disease which ruins vision slowly, with loss of central visual acuity in the late stages. Corticosteroid therapy *does not* prevent this progressive loss of vision. Systemic immunomodulatory therapy *does* prevent progressive loss of vision. The disease is probably triggered by some factor, such as a microbe, in genetically susceptible individuals.

This monograph was crafted by field experts and presenters during preparation for the Second International Symposium on Birdshot Retinochoroidopathy, held in Boston, Massachusetts on Saturday, September 28, 2013.

Acknowledgements

Choosing the topic for our annual Physician Education Conference was simple; the paucity of data on Birdshot Retinochoroidopathy, paired with the universal desire for more information from practitioners and patients alike forced the reprisal of this area of uveitis study. Birdshot Retinochoroidopathy is a rare and complicated disease, as this monograph explores on many levels, and as such, the care of these patients is judicious, almost tedious. Delivering this care would be absolutely impossible without the stellar team at the Massachusetts Eye Research and Surgery Institution (MERSI), including our technicians, laboratory staff, and office operations team. I am particularly grateful for the assistance of Scott Evans, Chief Operating Officer of MERSI and Treasurer of the Ocular Immunology and Uveitis Foundation (OIUF). Alison Justus, Director of Development of OIUF, deserves much praise for the logistical planning of this symposium down to the last detail. I also wish to acknowledge the Board of Directors of OIUF for their invaluable guidance throughout the planning of this conference. Drs. Ninani Kombo, H. Ayesha Hossain, and Pranav Patel, who are currently undergoing their fellowship training, represent the newest cohort of trained ocular immunologists; I am grateful for their assiduousness. I would like to express my gratitude to Jamie Lynne Metzinger and Bailey Wentworth for their completion of the painstaking tasks of gathering, editing, and reformatting the presentations and manuscripts of our presenters. Frances B. Foster deserves my special thanks for her presentation, and for her guidance as my partner at MERSI. Finally, my deepest gratitude is extended to this fantastic panel of presenters, who traveled from across the globe to gather, share insights, and report on the most recent advances in this blinding disease.

C. Stephen Foster

Chapter 1

Definition and Etiology

Antoine P. Brézin

*Birdshot retinochoroidopathy (BSRC) is a bilateral chronic posterior uveitis characterized by ovoid-shaped hypopigmented spots at the level of the choroid. Clinically based, internationally accepted, diagnostic criteria include the presence of these "birdshot lesions" and mild intraocular inflammation in both eyes. Birdshot retinochoroidopathy is also the disease with the strongest link to a class I HLA allele. At least 95% of patients are HLA-A29 carriers and, although not a recognized diagnostic criteria, a number of uveitis specialists restrict the diagnosis to HLA-A29 positive cases. The etiology of the disease is unknown. Birdshot retinochoroidopathy primarily affects patients of European descent. Among HLA-A29 subtypes, HLA-A*29:02 is most frequent in whites, while HLA-A*29:01 is more frequent in Asians. However, other factors, whether environmental and/or genetic, but most probably not HLA linked, are at play in the pathogenesis of the disease. In HLA-A*29:02 transgenic mice, a spontaneous posterior uveitis has been observed.*

Definition

Birdshot retinochoroidopathy is a bilateral chronic posterior uveitis named in 1980.[1] Previous descriptors of cases of posterior uveitis probably referred to the same entity and were previously labeled as retinochoroidopathy with "grains of rice" lesions, "salmon patch choroidopathy" or "vitiliginous chorioretinitis".[2] These various names refer to the particular "birdshot lesions", which are the hallmark of the disease. In their most typical presentation, these lesions are ovoid-shaped hypopigmented spots at the level of the choroid. Other features of the disease that were recognized in Ryan and Maumenee's original description of 13 cases of birdshot retinochoroidopathy were that the involved eyes were white, painless, with minimal anterior segment inflammation, but with particulate debris in the anterior and posterior vitreous. Profuse vascular leakage, with resultant retinal, macular and disk edema was observed.

An international workshop held in 2002 recommended diagnostic criteria for use in research regarding the disease.[3] Table 1 recapitulates these diagnostic criteria, which are based solely on clinical factors. The association of the disease with HLA-A29 discussed in the next section, was accepted as a supportive finding, but not as a diagnostic criterion. Hence, the diagnosis of birdshot retinochoroidopathy remains based on clinical findings and the observation of birdshot "spots" or "lesions" is the basis of the diagnosis. The international workshop recommendations were that at least three peripapillary lesions inferior or nasal to the optic disk in one eye were required for the diagnosis.

TABLE 1. *Birdshot Retinochoroidopathy: Diagnostic Criteria for Research Purposes*

Required characteristics

- Bilateral disease
- Presence of at least three peripapillary "birdshot lesions" inferior or nasal to the optic disk in one eye
- Low-grade anterior segment intraocular inflammation (defined as ≤ 1+cells in the anterior chamber)
- Low-grade vitreous inflammatory reaction (defined as ≤ 2+ vitreous haze)

Supportive findings

- HLA-A29 positivity
- Retinal vasculitis
- Cystoid macular edema

Exclusion criteria

- Keratic precipitates
- Posterior synechiae
- Presence of infectious, neoplastic, or other inflammatory diseases that can cause multifocal choroidal lesions

With permission from Levinson RD, Brézin AP, Rothova A, Accorinti M, Holland GN. Research criteria for the diagnosis of birdshot retinochoroidopathy: results of an international consensus conference. Am J Ophthalmol. 2006;141:185-7.

One of the main difficulties of the diagnosis lies in the spectrum of presentations of the spots. The typical lesions are ovoid with their main axis oriented toward the optic disc (Figure 1). However, some are round and they can be clearly seen on fundus examination while others can be limited to subtle depigmentations. Typical lesions are one-quarter to one-half disc diameters, but confluent lesions may yield larger areas of depigmentation that are difficult to recognize. Although the typical lesions are depigmented, their presentation may change over time and pigment or atrophy may replace the initial cream-colored spots. The typical location, or the most easily seen location of the spots, is nasal to the optic disc.

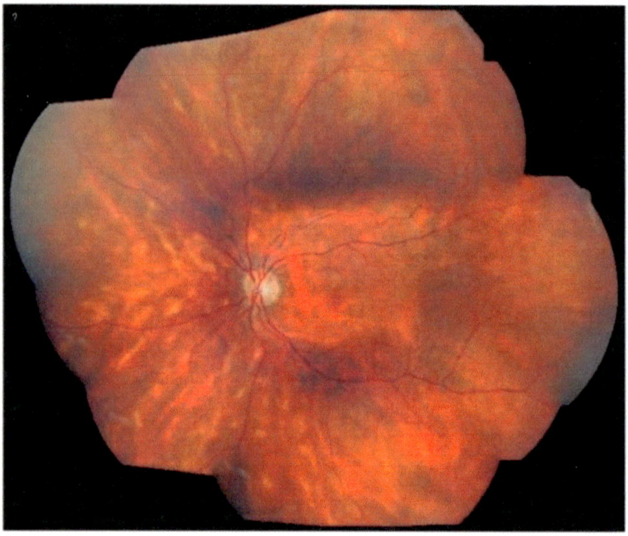

Figure 1.

However, involvement of the posterior pole inside the temporal arcade is also possible. The spots usually predominate in the mid-periphery, but may also extend to the equator. A standardized classification of the birdshot lesions according to their size, their number, their pigmentation and their localization has been suggested to help in the categorization of the various disease presentations and for the longitudinal follow-up of affected patients.[4] As illustrated in Figure 2a-b, spots clearly visible at the time of the diagnosis (2a) may disappear later (2b). Hence, if the diagnosis of the birdshot retinochoroidopathy is not made when spots are clearly visible, later presentations may not meet the definition commonly used for the disease. The disappearance of birdshot spots after treatment has been documented, but the effect of treatment on spots has not yet been assessed in large cohorts of patients.[5]

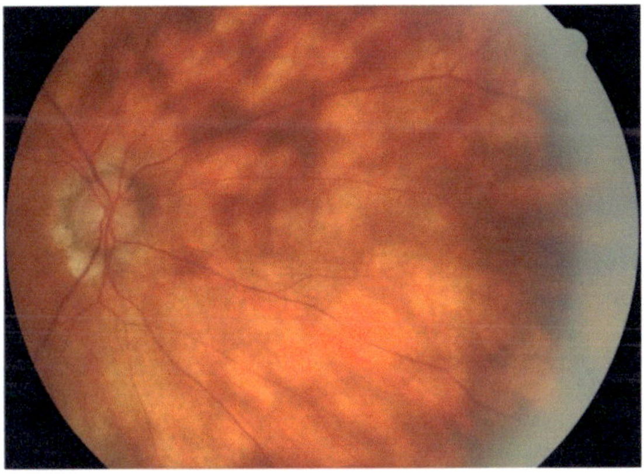

Figure 2a. *BSRC lesions visible at diagnosis*

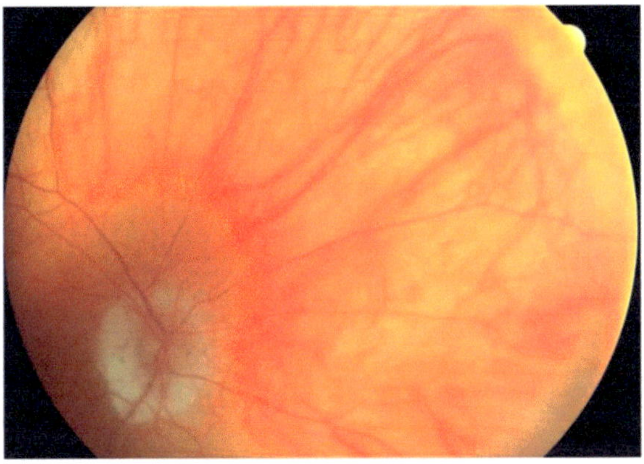

Figure 2b. *Lesions may seem to disappear*

Indocyanine green angiography has been suggested as a reliable method to detect spots.[6] However, it remains to be validated by a randomized assessment comparing indocyanine green angiography to color photographs for the detection of birdshot lesions.

Fluorescein angiography is useful in patients with birdshot retinochoroidopathy to assess disease activity. In active disease, angiographic findings include leakage of the retinal veins, macular edema and optic disk hyperfluorescence. These findings are not disease specific, but they require a careful examination of the fundus seeking subtle spots when birdshot lesions are not obvious.

Birdshot retinochoroidopathy and HLA-A29

One of the characteristics of birdshot retinochoroidopathy is its association with the HLA-A29 allele, which constitutes the strongest link between a disease and the class I HLA allele.[7] Linkage to HLA-A29 has been associated with a risk factor of 50 to 224 to develop birdshot retinochoroidopathy. Although a consensus has not been reached regarding HLA-A29 positivity as a requirement to make a diagnosis of birdshot retinochoroidopathy, the association is so strong that a number of uveitis specialists restrict the diagnosis to HLA-A29 positive cases.[8] Table 2 shows the prevalence of the HLA-A29 allele in series of patients with birdshot retinochoroidopathy.

The mechanism by which HLA-A29 confers a risk for birdshot retinochoroidopathy is a key question that remains unanswered. As with other associations between HLA class I antigens and diseases (HLA-B27 with spondylarthopathies and HLA-B51 with Behçet's disease), the physiopathogeny of these links have not been elucidated. Although the HLA-A29 allele is found with a greater frequency in the white

Table 2.

Reference			*Study Type*	*Number of Patients*	*Gender (%Female)*	*HLA-A29*
Authors	*Year*	*Journal*				
Shah *et al.*	2005	Surv Ophthalmol	Review	239	54.1	95.7
Oh KT *et al.*	2002	Am J Ophthalmol	Retrospective	19	52.6	100*(74)
Rothova *et al.*	2004	Ophthalmology	Retrospective	55	47.3	100
Kiss *et al.*	2005	Ophthalmology	Retrospective	28	50.0	96.4
Becker *et al.*	2005	Ocul Immunol Inflamm	Retrospective	11	54.5	100
Sobrin *et al.*	2005	Am J Ophthalmol	Retrospective	23	56.5	100
Holder et al.	2005	Br J Ophthalmol	Retrospective	18	NA	100*(89)
Monnet *et al.*	2006	Am J Ophthalmol	Cross-sectionnal	80	64.0	100
Thorne *et al.*	2008	Am J Ophthalmol	Retrospective	55	45.0	90* (43)
Rothova et al.	2011	Retina	Retrospective	76	64.5	100
Artornsombudh *et al.*	2013	Ophthalmology	Retrospective	22	77.3	95.4

* Some patients not tested for the presence of HLA-A29 (% of HLA-A29 positive among patients tested)

population (approximately 7%), this cannot totally account for the restriction of the disease to Caucasians.[9] Sequencing of the HLA class I region has now allowed the identification of more than 10 HLA-A29 subtypes. In Caucasians, HLA-A29*02 is approximately 20 times more prevalent than HLA-A29*01 and other subtypes are even more exceptional.[10] Previous reports had suggested that the disease could only be observed in A*2902 carriers.[11] In Asia where birdshot retinochoroidopathy is absent or extremely rare, HLA-A*2901 is the most frequent subtype. However, birdshot retinochoroidopathy has now been also observed in A*2901 Caucasian patients.[12] Therefore, other factors are sought, to explain why the disease is almost exclusively observed in Caucasians.

Hypotheses regarding the etiology of birdshot retinochoroidopathy

Other factors playing a role in the pathophysiology of the disease and not linked to the major histocompatibility complex are researched. These factors would either play a protective role in Asians, or favor an autoimmune reactivity in whites. Molecular mimicry with a microbial antigen has long been hypothesized to trigger diseases linked to an HLA allele. A few families of patients with birdshot retinochoroidopathy have been reported, which could point to additional genetic factors for disease susceptibility, but does not rule out an environmental effect.[13]

Two histological reports of birdshot retinochoroidopathy in HLA-A29 positive patients are available.[14,15] One was of the enucleated eye of a 55-year-old woman who has both birdshot retinochoroidopathy and ciliochoroidal melanoma. The other was of a 54 year-old man with birdshot retinochoroidopathy who died after a myocardial infarction. In both cases, multiple foci of predominantly lymphocytes were observed in the choroid, occasionally occupying the full choroidal thickness. The choroidal nodules of lymphocytes that showed the presence of CD3-positive cells also stained for CD4 or CD8.

Transgenic A29 mice develop spontaneous retinopathy with similarities to birdshot retinochoroidopathy.[16] Chorioretinal inflammation with retinal vasculitis, vitritis and papillitis with focal serous detachment of the retina and photoreceptor cell alterations were observed.[17] This model followed the report showing that rats transgenic for B27 develop a disorder resembling B27-associated human disease, with prominent intestinal, joint, skin, and male genital inflammatory lesions.[18] However, B27 transgenic rats raised in a germfree environment do not develop inflammatory intestinal or peripheral joint disease, whereas the skin and genital inflammatory lesions are unaffected by the germfree state.[19] As with B27-associated diseases, the environmental flora and in particular the commensal gut flora could play a role in the pathogenesis of birdshot retinochoroidopathy. Hence, the complex physiopathology of birdshot retinochoroidopathy could involve the HLA-A29 allele, other unknown genetic factors, as well as environmental factors.

References

1. Ryan SJ, Maumenee AE. Birdshot retinochoroidopathy. Am J Ophthalmol. 1980;89:31-45.
2. Shah KH, Levinson RD, Yu F, Goldhardt R, Gordon LK, Gonzales CR, Heckenlively JR, Kappel PJ, Holland GN. Birdshot retinochoroidopathy. Surv Ophthalmol. 2005;50:519-41.
3. Levinson RD, Brézin A, Rothova A, Accorinti M, Holland GN. Research criteria for the diagnosis of birdshot retinochoroidopathy: results of an international consensus conference. Am J Ophthalmol. 2006;141:185-7.
4. Monnet D, Brézin AP, Holland GN, Yu F, Mahr A, Gordon LK, Levinson RD. Longitudinal cohort study of patients with birdshot retinochoroidopathy. I. Baseline clinical characteristics. Am J Ophthalmol. 2006;141:135-42.
5. Leder HA, Galor A, Thorne JE, Jabs D. Disappearance of classic birdshot spots after immunosuppression with tacrolimus and mycophenolate mofetil. Br J Ophthalmol. 2008;92:291.
6. Fardeau C, Herbort CP, Kullmann N, Quentel G, LeHoang P. Indocyanine green angiography in birdshot retinochoroidopathy. Ophthalmology. 1999;106:1928-34.
7. Nussenblatt RB, Mittal KK, Ryan S, Green WR, Maumenee AE. Birdshot retinochoroidopathy associated with HLA-A29 antigen and immune responsiveness to retinal S-antigen. Am J Ophthalmol. 1982;94:147-58.
8. Monnet D, Brézin AP. Birdshot retinochoroidopathy. Curr Opin Ophthalmol. 2006;17:545-50.
9. Brézin AP, Monnet D, Cohen JH, Levinson RD. HLA-A29 and birdshot retinochoroidopathy. Ocul Immunol Inflamm. 2011;19:397-400.

10. Donvito B, Monnet D, Tabary T, Delair E, Vittier M, Réveil B, Chiquet C, Brézin AP, Cohen JH. A new HLA extended haplotype containing the A*2910 allele in birdshot retinochoroidopathy: susceptibility narrowed to the HLA molecule itself. Invest Ophthalmol Vis Sci. 2010 May;51(5):2525-8.
11. LeHoang P, Ozdemir N, Benhamou A, et al. HLA-A29.2 subtype associated with birdshot retinochoroidopathy. Am J Ophthalmol 1992;113:33-5.
12. Levinson RD, Rajalingam R, Park MS, et al. Human leukocyte antigen A29 subtypes associated with birdshot retinochoroidopathy. Am J Ophthalmol 2004;138:631-4.
13. Trinh L, Bodaghi B, Fardeau C, Monin C, Labetoulle M, Soubrane G, Lehoang P. Clinical features, treatment methods, and evolution of birdshot retinochoroidopathy in 5 different families. Am J Ophthalmol. 2009 Jun;147(6):1042-7.
14. Gaudio PA, Kaye DB, Crawford JB. Histopathology of birdshot retinochoroidopathy. Br J Ophthalmol. 2002;86:1439-41.
15. Pulido JS, Canal I, Salomão D, Kravitz D, Bradley E, Vile R. Histological findings of birdshot retinochoroidopathy in an eye with ciliochoroidal melanoma. Eye (Lond). 2012;26:862-5.
16. Szpak Y, Vieville JC, Tabary T, et al. Spontaneous retinopathy in HLA-A29 transgenic mice. Proc Natl Acad Sci U S A 2001;98:2572-6.
17. de Kozak Y, Camelo S, Pla M. Pathological aspects of spontaneous uveitis and retinopathy in HLA-A29 transgenic mice and in animal models of retinal autoimmunity: relevance to human pathologies. Ophthalmic Res. 2008;40:175-80.

18. Hammer RE, Maika SD, Richardson JA, Tang JP, Taurog JD. Spontaneous inflammatory disease in transgenic rats expressing HLA-B27 and human beta 2m: an animal model of HLA-B27-associated human disorders. Cell. 1990 30;63:1099-112.
19. Taurog JD, Richardson JA, Croft JT, Simmons WA, Zhou M, Fernández-Sueiro JL, Balish E, Hammer RE. The germfree state prevents development of gut and joint inflammatory disease in HLA-B27 transgenic rats. J Exp Med. 1994;180:2359-64.

Chapter 2

Epidemiology and Natural History

Albert T. Vitale

Birdshot retinochoroidopathy (BSRC) is an uncommon, bilateral, multifocal chorioretinal posterior uveitis occurring almost exclusively among whites of Northern European extraction with a mean age of onset of 53 years. It comprises 0.6%-1.5% of patients seen in tertiary referral centers for uveitis, or 6.0-7.9% of those with posterior uveitis. A slight female preponderance (54.1%) is present. There are no consistent systemic or ocular disease associations. Up to 96% of patients with BSRC are HLA-A29 positive, conferring significantly increased risk for the development of the disease; however, its presence alone is not diagnostic and does not explain the full spectrum of disease. Likewise, the differential distribution of HLA- subtypes (HLA-A29.2 and HLA-A29.1) does not explain the selective development of disease among whites with other genetic or acquired factors likely to be involved. The true natural history of BSRC is unknown; however, the preponderance of evidence suggests a chronic, progressive course marked by multiple inflammatory exacerbations associated with both central visual loss and global retinal dysfunction. Treatment with the early introduction of steroid-sparing immunomodulatory therapy (IMT) has therefore been advocated.

Since the initial description of birdshot retinochoroidopathy (BSRC) in 1980 by Ryan and Maumenee,[1] and subsequently by Gass in 1981,[2] there has been great interest in this disease, with nearly 100 publications in the literature on the various clinical and pathogenetic aspects of this entity. BSRC is an uncommon, bilateral, chronic, multifocal chorioretinal posterior uveitis comprising 0.6%-1.5% of patients seen in tertiary referral centers for uveitis, or 6.0-7.9% of those with posterior uveitis as reviewed by Shah and colleagues.[3] The largest series reported to date consists of 102 patients (203 eyes) collected from 14 European ophthalmology clinics between 1980 and 1986.[4] In the United States, Henderly and coworkers[5] reported only seven cases of BSRC among 600 patients (1.2%) referred to a specialized uveitis clinic while Gritz and Wong [6] identified only one case among 731,893 patients in a population-based study in Northern California. The emergence of BSRC as a "new" uveitic entity is reflected by Foster's experience in caring for 1,237 patients with uveitis between 1982 and 1992 in which 19 were identified as having this disease. This represents a prevalence of 7.9% of the 240 patients with posterior uveitis, the fifth most common entity of this subtype.[7] Between 1980 and 2003, 35 patients with BSRC were subsequently diagnosed and treated by the same physician.[8]

In contrast to many other uveitic entities in which the onset of disease is in younger age groups, BSRC typically occurs later in life at an average age of 53, with a range of between 15 and 79 years.[1-4,8-15] The reason for this shift towards middle age is unclear. BSRC is found almost exclusively among whites, with a higher incidence among those of

Northern European heritage, and is exceedingly uncommon among heavily pigmented ethnicities.[1,3,4,10-12,14,16,17] Overall, 54.1% of patients with BSRC are female (range 51% to 72.7%),[3] however, no significant sex predilection has been reported in some cohorts.[4,7,8,10,12,13,15,18,19]

BSRC is thought to be a predominantly ocular disease, developing in otherwise healthy patients without consistent systemic disease associations. However, careful medical history, examination, and review of symptoms may reveal associated cardiovascular disease, specifically systemic hypertension. Priem and Oosterhuis[4] noted an unusually high prevalence of vascular disease in their series of 102 patients with BSRC; 16 had systemic hypertension, 5 had coronary artery disease, 2 had suffered a cerebrovascular accident, and 3 had evidence of central retinal vein occlusion. Systemic hypertension was noted in 3 of our 19 patients with BSRC.[20] Among the National Eye Institute (NEI) cohort of BSRC patients, 75% had no significant systemic disease association, while 20% had idiopathic systemic hypertension, a prevalence well below that found among a similar patient population in the Framingham study.[14] Similarly, the prevalence of systemic hypertension was found to be 46% among 55 patients with BSCR followed for 5 years by Rothova and colleagues, a rate comparable to the estimated lifetime prevalence of 44% in the Dutch population.[12] Nearly one third of the patients reported by Monnet [9] and co-workers had systemic hypertension; however, treatment with cyclosporine in three of their patients is a potentially confounding factor. While it has been suggested that the presence of cardiovascular disease, specifically hypertension, may negatively influence the visual prognosis in

BSRC, there are no prospective data to corroborate this association. Other sporadic systemic associations among patients with funduscopic lesions typical of BSRC include case reports of autoimmune sensorineural hearing loss,[21] myelodysplasia syndrome,[22] and sarcoidosis.[4,23] Finally, while a 42% prevalence of atopic disease was reported in the cohort reported by Monnet and colleagues, this was similar to that previously noted for patients with BSRC, and so a definitive association or truly increased prevalence could not be established in the absence of an age-matched local control population.[9]

BSRC is unique in having the strongest association between an HLA and disease reported to date, suggesting a role for immune dysregulation in genetically predisposed individuals. Indeed, Pearlman and colleagues[24] reported an increased prevalence in systemic autoimmunity in both patients with white spot syndromes, including BSRC (25% of 16 individuals), as well as their first-and second-degree relatives. Specifically, the HLA-A29 phenotype is present in 85% to 96% of white patients with BSRC, with an overall estimate of 90%, compared to 7.7% of the general population.[4,15,25-28] The relative risk of developing BSRC in a patient bearing the HLA-A29 phenotype is between 50 and 224 times greater than that with other phenotypes.[4,25] While the sensitivity (96%) and specificity (93%) of the HLA-A29 phenotype in BSRC patients may be useful in suggesting this entity in the appropriate clinical context, it is neither sufficient nor necessary to make the diagnosis.[29,30] Feltkamp has calculated that the probability of a diagnosis of BSRC rises from 70% to 97% in HLA-A29-positive patients and drops from 70% to 8.5% in HLA-A29-negative individuals.[31] While this has led to some clinicians to screen patients with posterior uveitis for HLA-A29, Zamecki and Jabs point out that given the relative rarity of BSRC among patients with posterior uveitis (7%) and a 47% positive predictive value (PPV) of HLA-A29, the diagnosis of BSRC would be more often incorrect based on this test alone. Furthermore, even in a clinical context suggestive of the diagnosis, 4%-15% of BSRC patients are HLA-A29 negative.[32] While categorical screening may indeed be inappropriate, the negative predictive value of HLA-29 typing (99%) may be useful in patients with bilateral multifocal choroiditis and clinical features consistent with a diagnosis of BSRC, as a negative test should suggest an alternative diagnoses such as sarcoidosis or uveal lymphoma in the correct clinical context. While the disease has been reported to occur in monozygotic twins,[33] familial forms of BSRC are distinctly uncommon. Most recently, Trinh and colleagues reported 5 new families in which 2 members of each had BSRC; all were HLA-A29 positive.[34] While systematic examination in relatives of patients with BSRC may not be warranted, this uncommon presentation should be kept in mind in the differential diagnosis of atypical forms of retinitis pigmentosa.

A peculiar aspect of the epidemiology of BSRC is its essential restriction to the Caucasian population. Sequencing of the Class I region has revealed more than 20 HLA-A29 subtypes, the most common being HLA-A29.2, and HLA-A29.1, the frequency and distribution of each varying with ethnicity.[35] Among HLA-A29 positive healthy white patients Northern European extraction, the HLA-A29.2 subtype is present in approximately 80-100% whereas the

HLA-A29.1 subtype is found more commonly among populations from Southeast Asia where BSRC is absent or extremely rare.[19] Indeed, in their analysis of a subgroup of 33 white French patients with BSRC, Le Hoang and colleagues[15] found the HLA-A29.2 subtype in all subjects (100%). De Waal and coworkers,[19] on the other hand, found that the distribution of HLA-A29 subtypes in their group of 20 Northern European patients with birdshot retinochoroidopathy did not differ from that found among healthy controls.[19] Whereas both subtypes were found among BSRC patients, HLA-29.2 was more frequently identified because of its overwhelming prevalence (90%) in this particular study population. While case reports exist among Hispanic[14] and African American patients in the USA,[36] and from Japan,[37] the disease is virtually nonexistent in Asia and the Indian subcontinent. The differential distribution of HLA-A29.2 and HLA-A29.1 among whites and Asians respectively has been cited as an explanation for the selective development of BSRC in patients for Northern European descent, with HLA-A29.2 thought to confer significant risk for the development of disease, while a "resistance motif" has been invoked in association with HLA-A29.1.[38,39] In the United States, the gene frequency of HLA-29.2 is 4.34% in whites, 3.57% in African Americans, and 4.91% in Hispanics and 0.42% in Asian Americans.[40] Corresponding gene frequencies for HLA-A29.1 include 0.19% in whites, 0.21% in Hispanics and 0.125% in Asian Americans. The low frequency of HLA-A29.2 in Asian Americans may partially explain the paucity of reported cases in this group; however, it does not among African Americans and Hispanics who appear strikingly protected from the disease.

Recently, high resolution DNA typing of HLA-A29 among 20 patients with BSRC failed to support a protective role for HLA-A29.1 as both HLA-A29.1 and HLA-A29.2 were associated with disease.[28] Likewise, HLA-A29.1 has been reported in 2 white patients with a clinical diagnosis of BSRC; the HLA-A29.1 haplotype for white patients and Asian healthy subjects being identical, together with HLA-A29.1 and HLA-A29.2 complotypes. In addition, susceptibility to BSRC seemed to be located in the microsatellites near the locus HLA-A, and not on the HLA-A29 molecule itself.[35,41] While disease susceptibility appears to be associated with the HLA-A29 molecule, irrespective of subtype, these data suggest that heretofore unidentified genetic or acquired factors, not linked to the major histocompatibility complex (MHC), are either protective in Asians, Hispanics and Africans or conversely, trigger autoimmune reactivity in whites where the prevalence of BSRC in the HLA-A29 population remains low.

Levinson and colleagues[42] have reported that specific allelic combinations of the killer cell immunoglobulin-like receptor (KIR) gene, which encode for inhibitory and activating receptors expressed on human natural killer (NK) cells and some T cells, including CD8 + T lymphocytes. Both are important in innate and adaptive immunity and confer significant risk for the development of disease in HLA-A29 positive patients with BSRC while other compound genotypes were relatively protective. These genes may contribute to the pathogenesis of BSRC by activating NK cells and T-cell subsets against intraocular self-antigens.

The natural history of BSRC is unknown. Some investigators have reported a self-limiting course in 20%[14] and believe that BSRC has a tendency to stabilize over a 3-to 4-year period and go into remission.[16] The preponderance of experience suggests a chronic, progressive course, marked by multiple exacerbations and remissions that may extend over a period of decades, resulting in atrophic changes in the retina and optic nerve and a guarded visual prognosis.[1,2,4,12,13,20,25] Some patients may have relatively good visual acuity on presentation, but as many as 20% may experience a reduction in visual acuity of three Snellen lines or more, with greater than one third of such eyes reaching a level of 20/200 or worse in at least one eye.[1,2,4] Rothova and colleagues[12] noted strong associations between visual acuity at onset and visual outcome at 5 and 10 years with the number of affected eyes with VA ≤ 20/200 increasing from 9 of 108 (8%) at onset to 22 of 73 (30%) at 5 years and 19 of 49 (39%) at 10 years of follow-up. Most recently, Thorne and associates[10] reported the incidence rates on follow-up vision loss to ≤20/50 and to ≤20/200 to be 13% and 4% per eye-year (EY) respectively among 44 patients with BSRC followed for a decade. There was a 20%, 5 year cumulative incidence of VA ≤20/200, corroborating previous observations by Rothova. Longer duration of disease was associated with poorer visual outcomes and a higher proportion of structural ocular complications independent of previous oral corticosteroid therapy.

Central visual loss is most commonly the result of CME, occurring at a rate of 10% per eye/year (EY).[3,10,12] However, chronic, progressive retinal dysfunction, as measured by perimetry and electroretinography, together with macular and optic nerve atrophy, may occur even in the absence of clinically evident CME or vitritis, resulting not only in loss of central vision, but also in global retinal function.[13] Indeed, progressive loss of visual field and deterioration of ERG parameters may occur even in the presence of relatively stable visual acuity.

Given the uncertain natural history and visual prognosis, and the fact that the usual proxy markers for intraocular inflammation (anterior, vitreous cell and haze) may not always be evident, we and others have advocated an aggressive treatment approach with the early introduction of steroid-sparing immunomodulatory therapy (IMT) for patients with BSRC. The presence of inflammation, whether manifest by obvious CME or vitritis, more subtle retinal or choroidal vasculitis as seen on FA or ICG angiography, or changes in visual field or ERG parameters, rather than an arbitrary level of visual acuity, guide our therapeutic decisions in an effort to limit permanent ocular structural damage and preserve visual function.

References

1. Ryan SJ, Maumenee AE. Birdshot retinochoroidopathy. *Am J Ophthalmol.* Jan 1980;89(1):31-45.
2. Gass JD. Vitiliginous chorioretinitis. *Arch Ophthalmol.* Oct 1981;99(10):1778-1787.
3. Shah KH, Levinson RD, Yu F, et al. Birdshot retinochoroidopathy. *Surv Ophthalmol.* Nov-Dec 2005;50(6):519-541.
4. Priem HA, Oosterhuis JA. Birdshot retinochoroidopathy: clinical characteristics and evolution. *Br J Ophthalmol.* Sep 1988;72(9):646-659.
5. Henderly DE, Genstler AJ, Smith RE, Rao NA. Changing patterns of uveitis. *Am J Ophthalmol.* Feb 15 1987;103(2):131-136.
6. Gritz DC, Wong IG. Incidence and prevalence of uveitis in Northern California; the Northern California Epidemiology of Uveitis Study. *Ophthalmology.* Mar 2004;111(3):491-500; discussion 500.
7. Rodriguez A, Calonge M, Pedroza-Seres M, et al. Referral patterns of uveitis in a tertiary eye care center. *Arch Ophthalmol.* May 1996;114(5):593-599.
8. Kiss S, Ahmed M, Letko E, Foster CS. Long-term follow-up of patients with birdshot retinochoroidopathy treated with corticosteroid-sparing systemic immunomodulatory therapy. *Ophthalmology.* Jun 2005;112(6):1066-1071.
9. Monnet D, Brezin AP, Holland GN, et al. Longitudinal cohort study of patients with birdshot retinochoroidopathy. I. Baseline clinical characteristics. *Am J Ophthalmol.* Jan 2006;141(1):135-142.

10. Thorne JE, Jabs DA, Peters GB, Hair D, Dunn JP, Kempen JH. Birdshot retinochoroidopathy: ocular complications and visual impairment. *Am J Ophthalmol.* Jul 2005;140(1):45-51.
11. Becker MD, Wertheim MS, Smith JR, Rosenbaum JT. Long-term follow-up of patients with birdshot retinochoroidopathy treated with systemic immunosuppression. *Ocul Immunol Inflamm.* Jul-Aug 2005;13(4):289-293.
12. Rothova A, Berendschot TT, Probst K, van Kooij B, Baarsma GS. Birdshot retinochoroidopathy: long-term manifestations and visual prognosis. *Ophthalmology.* May 2004;111(5):954-959.
13. Oh KT, Christmas NJ, Folk JC. Birdshot retinochoroidopathy: long term follow-up of a chronically progressive disease. *Am J Ophthalmol.* May 2002;133(5):622-629.
14. Gasch AT, Smith JA, Whitcup SM. Birdshot retinochoroidopathy. *Br J Ophthalmol.* Feb 1999;83(2):241-249.
15. LeHoang P, Ozdemir N, Benhamou A, et al. HLA-A29.2 subtype associated with birdshot retinochoroidopathy. *Am J Ophthalmol.* Jan 15 1992;113(1):33-35.
16. Fuerst DJ, Tessler HH, Fishman GA, Yokoyama MM, Wyhinny GJ, Vygantas CM. Birdshot retinochoroidopathy. *Arch Ophthalmol.* Feb 1984;102(2):214-219.
17. Kaplan HJ, Aaberg TM. Birdshot retinochoroidopathy. *Am J Ophthalmol.* Dec 1980;90(6):773-782.
18. Brucker AJ, Deglin EA, Bene C, Hoffman ME. Subretinal choroidal neovascularization in birdshot retinochoroidopathy. *Am J Ophthalmol.* Jan 15 1985;99(1):40-44.

19. de Waal LP, Lardy NM, van der Horst AR, et al. HLA-A29 subtypes and birdshot retinochoroidopathy. *Immunogenetics.* 1992;35(1):51-53.
20. Vitale AT, Rodriguez A, Foster CS. Low-dose cyclosporine therapy in the treatment of birdshot retinochoroidopathy. *Ophthalmology.* May 1994;101(5):822-831.
21. Heaton JM, Mills RP. Sensorineural hearing loss associated with birdshot retinochoroidopathy. *Arch Otolaryngol Head Neck Surg.* Jun 1993;119(6):680-681.
22. Noble KG, Greenberg J. Appearance of birdshot retinochoroidopathy in a patient with myelodysplasia syndrome. *Am J Ophthalmol.* Jan 1998;125(1):108-109.
23. Yoshioka T, Yoshioka H, Tanaka F. [Birdshot retinochoroidopathy as a new ocular sign of the sarcoidosis]. *Nippon Ganka Gakkai Zasshi.* 1983;87(4):283-288.
24. Pearlman RB, Golchet PR, Feldmann MG, et al. Increased prevalence of autoimmunity in patients with white spot syndromes and their family members. *Arch Ophthalmol.* Jul 2009;127(7):869-874.
25. Nussenblatt RB, Mittal KK, Ryan S, Green WR, Maumenee AE. Birdshot retinochoroidopathy associated with HLA-A29 antigen and immune responsiveness to retinal S-antigen. *Am J Ophthalmol.* Aug 1982;94(2):147-158.
26. Oruc S, Kaplan AD, Galen M, Kaplan HJ. Uveitis referral pattern in a Midwest University Eye Center. *Ocul Immunol Inflamm.* Dec 2003;11(4):287-298.
27. Baarsma GS, Priem HA, Kijlstra A. Association of birdshot retinochoroidopathy and HLA-A29 antigen. *Curr Eye Res.* 1990;9 Suppl:63-68.

28. Levinson RD, Rajalingam R, Park MS, et al. Human leukocyte antigen A29 subtypes associated with birdshot retinochoroidopathy. *Am J Ophthalmol.* Oct 2004;138(4):631-634.
29. Feltkamp TE. Ophthalmological significance of HLA associated uveitis. *Eye (Lond).* 1990;4 (Pt 6):839-844.
30. Levinson RD, Brezin A, Rothova A, Accorinti M, Holland GN. Research criteria for the diagnosis of birdshot retinochoroidopathy: results of an international consensus conference. *Am J Ophthalmol.* Jan 2006;141(1):185-187.
31. Feltkamp TE. HLA and uveitis. *Int Ophthalmol.* Oct 1990;14(5-6):327-333.
32. Zamecki KJ, Jabs DA. HLA typing in uveitis: use and misuse. *Am J Ophthalmol.* Feb 2010;149(2):189-193 e182.
33. Fich M, Rosenberg T. Birdshot retinochoroidopathy in monozygotic twins. *Acta Ophthalmol (Copenh).* Oct 1992;70(5):693-697.
34. Trinh L, Bodaghi B, Fardeau C, et al. Clinical features, treatment methods, and evolution of birdshot retinochoroidopathy in 5 different families. *Am J Ophthalmol.* Jun 2009;147(6):1042-1047, 1047 e1041.
35. Donvito B, Monnet D, Tabary T, et al. Different HLA class IA region complotypes for HLA-A29.2 and -A29.1 antigens, identical in birdshot retinochoroidopathy patients or healthy individuals. *Invest Ophthalmol Vis Sci.* Sep 2005;46(9):3227-3232.
36. Barondes MJ, Fastenberg DM, Schwartz PL, Rosen DA. Peripheral retinal neovascularization in birdshot retinochoroidopathy. *Ann Ophthalmol.* Aug 1989;21(8):306-308.

37. Saito W, Yamamoto S, Mitamura Y, Takeuchi S. [Birdshot retinochoroidopathy--a case report and a case study in Japanese patients]. *Nippon Ganka Gakkai Zasshi.* Apr 2002;106(4):229-235.
38. Tabary T, Lehoang P, Betuel H, et al. Susceptibility to birdshot retinochoroidopathy is restricted to the HLA-A29.2 subtype. *Tissue Antigens.* Oct 1990;36(4):177-179.
39. Tabary T, Prochnicka-Chalufour A, Cornillet P, Lehoang P, Betuel H, Cohen JH. [HLA-A29 sub-types and "Birdshot" choroido-retinopathy susceptibility: a possible "resistance motif" in the HLA-A29.1 molecule]. *C R Acad Sci III.* 1991;313(13):599-605.
40. Cao K, Hollenbach J, Shi X, Shi W, Chopek M, Fernandez-Vina MA. Analysis of the frequencies of HLA-A, B, and C alleles and haplotypes in the five major ethnic groups of the United States reveals high levels of diversity in these loci and contrasting distribution patterns in these populations. *Hum Immunol.* Sep 2001;62(9):1009-1030.
41. Donvito B, Monnet D, Tabary T, et al. A new HLA extended haplotype containing the A*2910 allele in birdshot retinochoroidopathy: susceptibility narrowed to the HLA molecule itself. *Invest Ophthalmol Vis Sci.* May 2010;51(5):2525-2528.
42. Levinson RD, Du Z, Luo L, et al. Combination of KIR and HLA gene variants augments the risk of developing birdshot retinochoroidopathy in HLA-A*29-positive individuals. *Genes Immun.* Apr 2008;9(3):249-258.

Chapter 3

Evidence of Autoimmunity

Breno R. Lima, H. Nida Sen, Robert B. Nussenblatt

Birdshot retinochoroidopathy is an inflammatory disease restricted to the eye, with a strong association to HLA-A29. Retinal autoimmunity and genetic predisposition play a major role in the pathogenesis of this rare disease. Further understanding of immune mechanisms involved in its pathophysiology may lead to targeted treatment strategies.

Birdshot retinochoroidopathy (BSRC) is a potentially blinding inflammatory disease that affects the posterior segment of the eye, characterized by multiple bilateral hypopigmented retinal pigment epithelial and choroidal lesions radiating from the optic nerve, which become more apparent with disease progression, vitritis, and retinal vascular leakage. BSRC generally presents in middle age, affecting mainly Caucasians, with the average age of presentation around 50 years.[1,2]

Patients usually experience nyctalopia, photopsias, dyschromatopsia and progressive visual decline. Without treatment, retinal function typically deteriorates over time.[1]

Although the pathogenesis of BSRC is not completely elucidated, studies have demonstrated that retinal autoimmunity and genetic predisposition play a major role in the manifestation of this rare disease.[3]

Genetic and autoimmune factors in birdshot retinochoroidopathy

Several inflammatory disorders are associated with the presence of specific genes, particularly with the human leukocyte antigen (HLA) genes on the major histocompatibility complex of chromosome 6. Experimental studies have demonstrated that a specific human major histocompatibility complex allele (HLA-A29) confers susceptibility to BSRC.[4] HLA-A29 has been observed in more than 95% of patients with BSRC compared to 7% in the general population. The relative risk of developing BSRC among

HLA-A29 positive individuals has been estimated to be between 50 – 224, one of the highest reported for any human disease.[5] However, contrasting to other HLA-associated diseases, there is no known predominant extraocular manifestation.[6]

Experimental and clinical evidence suggest an autoimmune etiology for BSRC, involving T lymphocyte mediated responses with a strong association to HLA-A29.[6] Two subtypes of HLA-A29 have been documented, HLA-A29.1 and HLA-A29.2. These subtypes have a single amino acid difference. A29.2 subtype is considerably more common.[7] One hypothesis advocates that self-peptides, associated with HLA-A29, may have a role in positive selection of developing thymocytes, specific for particular autoantigens in the choroid and retina.[4] Few reports have described the histopathological analysis of eyes from patients with BSCR.[3,8,9] Aggregation of lymphocytes at various levels of the choroid, around the retinal vasculature and in the prelaminar optic nerve head have been documented.[8] Pulido et al. reported the histological findings of BSRC in an eye with ciliochoroidal melanoma. Presence of nodular lymphocytic infiltrates in the choroid, with a mixture of T cells (both CD4+ and CD8+ cells), a few CD20+ B cells and rare CD68+ histiocytes were noted in the enucleated eye, separate from the melanoma.[9] A diffuse, chronic granulomatous inflammation of the retina and choroid, with diffuse retinal atrophy, has been described in a HLA-A29 antigen negative patient with BSRC.[3]

A few studies have shown the important role of T helper 17 (Th17) cells in autoimmune diseases, including rheumatoid arthritis, Crohn's disease and HLA-B27-associated ankylosing spondylitis.[10,11] These cells produce interleukin IL-17.[12] Elevated levels of IL-17 have been documented in peripheral blood mononuclear cells during active uveitis and scleritis, and with decreased levels following treatment.[13] Kuiper and associates, using a multiplex immunoassay, demonstrated that IL-17 and IL-2, and proinflammatory mediators IL-1β, IL-6 and TNF-α were elevated in the aqueous humor of BSRC patients, supporting the role of a Th17 cell-mediated inflammatory response localized to the eye.[14] IL-2 is a known growth factor for T lymphocytes, including Th17 cells.[13,15] In addition, IL-6 has a role in the development of Th17 cells, forcing naive T lymphocytes to express IL-17 and to become Th17 cells.[12] IL-6 can also promote IL-17 production by natural killer cells.[16] Newly diagnosed BSRC patients with active disease naïve to systemic immunosuppressive therapy (IMT) have been reported to display a serum cytokine profile with significantly elevated levels of TGF-β1, IL-21 and IL-23, which are known to be necessary to Th17 cell differentiation and production of IL-17.[6]

Recent evidence has suggested that regulatory T lymphocytes (Tregs) may have effects in the regulation of ocular self-tolerance in patients with BSRC. In a pilot study by Foster et al. the percentage of CD4+ CD25+ FOXP3+ Tregs was significantly lower in BSRC patients compared with controls.[4]

The discovery of killer cell immunoglobulin-like receptors (KIR) led to several studies implicating KIRs in autoimmune diseases. They are key receptors of human natural killer (NK) cells. CD8+ cytotoxic T lymphocytes and CD4+ $CD28^{null}$ also express KIRs.[17] A strong association has been noted between the development of BSRC and the genes KIR2DS2, 2DS3 and 2DS4, which are the same genes implicated in other autoimmune diseases.[17,18] Although the direct role of NK cells in BSRC is unclear, it is possible that these genes influence the activation of NK cells and cytotoxic T cells to respond to intraocular self-antigens.[17]

Lymphocytes from patients with BSRC demonstrate an in vitro cell-mediated response to retinal antigens, particularly the retinal S-antigen.[3] Jobin et al. found that in vitro positivity to S-antigen, using lymphocyte proliferation or basophil degranulation test, was significantly more frequent in the period preceding a relapse of ocular inflammation.[19]

Animal models have corroborated the concept that immune mechanisms play a major role in BSRC. Monkeys immunized with the retinal S-antigen display features similar to those seen in humans with this disease. Aging HLA-A29 transgenic mice developed spontaneous retinopathy with features similar to BSRC.[20] A study by de Kozak et al. demonstrated similar findings. HLA-A29 transgenic mice showed photoreceptor alterations, with retinal vasculopathy and papillitis and inflammatory lesions in the retina and choroid. The fact that HLA molecules play a central role in antigen-presenting cells strongly suggests that the HLA-A29 molecule itself is involved in the pathogenesis of

BSRC, along with retinal autoimmunity, which perpetuates intraocular inflammation that was already initiated.[20,21]

Some authors have proposed that an infection could also have influence in the pathogenesis of BSRC, by causing an immune response to the organism itself or to antigens through molecular mimicry, facilitated by the presentation of self-antigens by the HLA-A29 molecule.[20-22] *Borrelia burgdorferi* has been one of the suspects. However, this agent has never been found morphologically in the retina of patients with BSRC. Further studies are needed to investigate this connection.[22]

Birdshot retinochoroidopathy may have guarded prognosis regarding visual function in a large proportion of cases, if not treated early. Several immunomodulatory regimens have been explored in the management of BSRC, including cyclosporine, mycophenolate mofetil, and other IMT agents, either alone or in combination. They have been reported to induce control of inflammation in the majority of cases and reduce visual impairment and vision field loss, further supporting the role of autoimmunity in this disease.[23-27]

In summary, BSRC is an inflammatory autoimmune disease with a strong association to HLA-A29. Further investigation of the immune mechanisms related to the pathogenesis of this rare disease may lead to the development of targeted treatment strategies.

References

1. Kiss S, Anzaar F, Stephen Foster C. Birdshot retinochoroidopathy. Int Ophthalmol Clin 2006;46:39-55.
2. Monnet D, Brezin AP. Birdshot retinochoroidopathy. Curr Opin Ophthalmol 2006;17:545-50.
3. Nussenblatt RB, Mittal KK, Ryan S, Green WR, Maumenee AE. Birdshot retinochoroidopathy associated with HLA-A29 antigen and immune responsiveness to retinal S-antigen. American journal of ophthalmology 1982;94:147-58.
4. Foster CS, Siddique SS, Amorese L, Mulki L, Suelves A. Regulatory T cells in blood of patients with birdshot retinochoroidopathy. Ophthalmology 2013;120:430 e1.
5. Lima BR, Nussenblatt RB, Sen HN. Pharmacogenetics of drugs used in the treatment of ocular inflammatory diseases. Expert Opin Drug Metab Toxicol 2013;9:875-82.
6. Yang P, Foster CS. Interleukin 21, Interleukin 23, and Transforming Growth Factor beta1 in HLA-A29-Associated Birdshot Retinochoroidopathy. American journal of ophthalmology 2013.
7. Boisgerault F, Khalil I, Tieng V, et al. Definition of the HLA-A29 peptide ligand motif allows prediction of potential T-cell epitopes from the retinal soluble antigen, a candidate autoantigen in birdshot retinopathy. Proc Natl Acad Sci U S A 1996;93:3466-70.
8. Gaudio PA, Kaye DB, Crawford JB. Histopathology of birdshot retinochoroidopathy. Br J Ophthalmol 2002;86:1439-41.

9. Pulido JS, Canal I, Salomao D, Kravitz D, Bradley E, Vile R. Histological findings of birdshot retinochoroidopathy in an eye with ciliochoroidal melanoma. Eye (Lond) 2012;26:862-5.
10. Holtta V, Klemetti P, Sipponen T, et al. IL-23/IL-17 immunity as a hallmark of Crohn's disease. Inflamm Bowel Dis 2008;14:1175-84.
11. McInnes IB, Schett G. Cytokines in the pathogenesis of rheumatoid arthritis. Nat Rev Immunol 2007;7:429-42.
12. Miossec P, Korn T, Kuchroo VK. Interleukin-17 and type 17 helper T cells. N Engl J Med 2009;361:888-98.
13. Amadi-Obi A, Yu CR, Liu X, et al. TH17 cells contribute to uveitis and scleritis and are expanded by IL-2 and inhibited by IL-27/STAT1. Nat Med 2007;13:711-8.
14. Kuiper JJ, Mutis T, de Jager W, de Groot-Mijnes JD, Rothova A. Intraocular interleukin-17 and proinflammatory cytokines in HLA-A29-associated birdshot retinochoroidopathy. American journal of ophthalmology 2011;152:177-82 e1.
15. Gillis S, Watson J. Biochemical and biological characterization of lymphocyte regulatory molecules. V. Identification of an interleukin 2-producing human leukemia T cell line. J Exp Med 1980;152:1709-19.
16. Passos ST, Silver JS, O'Hara AC, Sehy D, Stumhofer JS, Hunter CA. IL-6 promotes NK cell production of IL-17 during toxoplasmosis. J Immunol 2010;184:1776-83.
17. Levinson RD, Du Z, Luo L, et al. Combination of KIR and HLA gene variants augments the risk of developing birdshot retinochoroidopathy in HLA-A*29-positive individuals. Genes Immun 2008;9:249-58.

18. Yen JH, Lin CH, Tsai WC, et al. Killer cell immunoglobulin-like receptor gene's repertoire in rheumatoid arthritis. Scandinavian journal of rheumatology 2006;35:124-7.
19. Jobin D, Thillaye B, de Kozak Y, Sainte-Laudy J, Faure JP, Le Hoang P. Severe retinochoroidopathy: variations of humoral and cellular immunity to S-antigen in a longitudinal study. Curr Eye Res 1990;9 Suppl:91-6.
20. Szpak Y, Vieville JC, Tabary T, et al. Spontaneous retinopathy in HLA-A29 transgenic mice. Proc Natl Acad Sci U S A 2001;98:2572-6.
21. de Kozak Y, Camelo S, Pla M. Pathological aspects of spontaneous uveitis and retinopathy in HLA-A29 transgenic mice and in animal models of retinal autoimmunity: relevance to human pathologies. Ophthalmic Res 2008;40:175-80.
22. Holak HM, Szymaniec S, Holak SA. The pathogenesis of birdshot retinochoroidopathy. Surv Ophthalmol 2006;51:446-7; author reply 7.
23. Thorne JE, Jabs DA, Kedhar SR, Peters GB, Dunn JP. Loss of visual field among patients with birdshot retinochoroidopathy. American journal of ophthalmology 2008;145:23-8.
24. Thorne JE, Jabs DA, Peters GB, Hair D, Dunn JP, Kempen JH. Birdshot retinochoroidopathy: ocular complications and visual impairment. American journal of ophthalmology 2005;140:45-51.
25. Cervantes-Castaneda RA, Gonzalez-Gonzalez LA, Cordero-Coma M, Yilmaz T, Foster CS. Combined therapy of cyclosporine A and mycophenolate mofetil for the treatment of birdshot retinochoroidopathy: a 12-month follow-up. Br J Ophthalmol 2013;97:637-43.

26. Nussenblatt RB, Palestine AG, Chan CC. Cyclosporin A therapy in the treatment of intraocular inflammatory disease resistant to systemic corticosteroids and cytotoxic agents. American journal of ophthalmology 1983;96:275-82.
27. Artornsombudh P, Gevorgyan O, Payal A, Siddique SS, Foster CS. Infliximab treatment of patients with birdshot retinochoroidopathy. Ophthalmology 2013;120:588-92.

Chapter 4

Immunogenetics

Ralph D. Levinson

*Birdshot retinochoroidopathy (BSRC) has an association with the HLA-A*29 allele that is sufficiently strong for HLA typing to be used as a diagnostic tool. A negative HLA-A29 test minimally suggests that other diagnoses should be considered, although HLA-A29 negative BSRC has been reported. The HLA-A*2902 subtype is the most common, but HLA-A*2901 and A*2910 have been reported in patients with BSRC. HLA-A*29 positivity, however, is not sufficient for the development of BSRC; in fact the disease is rare even in A29 positive individuals, and in certain populations in which A*29 is found BSRC is exceedingly rare. Strong associations have also been described with genes for killer immunoglobulin receptors as well as HLA-Bw4, particularly HLA-B44. The latter gene may be present due to linkage disequilibrium, but there is evidence for selection due to interaction with KIRs. Clearly more genes (and environmental factors) remain to be elucidated.*

Birdshot retinochoroidopathy (BSRC) is fascinating from the point of view of immunogenetics. The association of BSRC and HLA-A29 is one of the strongest in medicine. Of course the presence of the HLA-A*29 allele is not sufficient to by itself to cause disease. It is likely that being HLA-A29 positive and Caucasian, without a family history of BSRC, confers a risk of developing BSRC that is less than one in a thousand, probably closer to one in five thousand, although specific data are not available. The presence of the disease in families suggests additional genetic factors as well. In addition, African Americans have about half the rate of HLA-A29 positivity that Caucasians do, but the disease is exceedingly rare in African Americans, if it occurs at all. I have only heard anecdotally of a few cases, and no convincing case has been published.

In fact, BSRC may be only disease where HLA typing genuinely plays a diagnostic role; it certainly is unique in ophthalmology. Even the association of HLA-B27 in acute anterior uveitis is not as strong as that for HLA-A29 and BSRC; the HLA-B27 status of a patient with acute anterior uveitis is more important for prognosis and implications for systemic involvement than diagnosis per se. HLA-A29 testing does have sufficient predictive positivity and negativity to be considered useful in the work up of the patient. Of course as 7-8% of Caucasians are HLA-A29 positive, patients with other diseases can also be HLA-A29 positive; the predictive positivity of the test is not 100%. Conversely some patients that have all the clinical features of BSRC have been HLA-29 negative, even with the latest techniques and repeated testing. In a published analysis done by Zamecki and Jabs[1] the positive predictive value of HLA-

A29 was only 0.47; the negative predictive value, however, was 0.99! However when patients with BSRC were compared to multifocal choroiditis and panuveitis the predictive positive and negative values were found to be 0.92 and .90 respectively.[1] The data employed for this study was a group of patients with a lower rate of HLA-A29 positivity (90% in the analysis but 96% in the literature) than the rate in the published literature as well as the experience of others (for example at UCLA or Hôpital Cochin, Paris, France). This suggests that the true predictive positive and negative values may be even higher, strongly supporting HLA-A29 as a diagnostic tool, particularly in the setting of a negative test. If the patient is negative for HLA-A29, it at least raises a "red flag" that other diagnoses such as sarcoidosis or even lymphoma need to be considered. A problem in the past was false negative HLA-A29 testing, leading to a delay in diagnosis for some patients. Most laboratories now use DNA based methods rather than serologic HLA testing and thus false negative testing is less common.

There has been some controversy as to whether specific HLA-A29 subtypes play different roles in conferring risk for BSRC. There are now more than 20 subtypes of HLA-A29 described. A difference between risks conferred by HLA subtypes is plausible and has been found for HLA associations with other types of uveitis. The subtype found most often in patients with BSRC is the HLA-A*2902 subtype, which is also more common than other HLA-A29 subtypes. The next most common HLA-A29 subtype in Caucasians is HLA-A*2901, which is only found in 5% or less of HLA-A29 positive individuals. We reported a relatively high rate of HLA-A*2901 in our patients with

BSRC, so despite some earlier studies to the contrary, at least regarding these two subtypes, there is little reason to think there is much difference regarding risk for BSRC.[2] Further, the HLA-A*2902 subtype is also more common in Hispanics and African Americans, so this would not explain the much lower incidence of disease in these populations. In fact, the group at Hôpital Cochin found two patients with a new extended HLA-A*2910 haplotype; they also presented evidence that it is the HLA-29 gene and not the surrounding linked genes in these haplotypes, that confers risk.[3,4]

Another HLA type, Bw4, specifically HLA-B44, has also been found to be associated with BSRC. It is known that HLA-B44 is in linkage disequilibrium with HLA-A29, and so it is likely that HLA-A29 is the driving force behind this association. Nonetheless, in a study done in collaboration with Drs. Brezin and Monnet from Hôpital Cochin and Dr. Jacques Cohen from Reims we found that the subtype of HLA-B44 found in patients differed from French controls.[5] The Bw4 T80 subtype that primarily consists of HLA-B44 in BSRC patients that was found in patients was one that reacts more strongly with killer immunoglobulin receptors (KIRs). The KIR gene 3DL1 and Bw4 T80 combination was found to be strongly associated with disease with an odds ratio of 10.47, one of the highest for any KIR association for any disease (p value= 0.000016).[5] HLA-B44, KIRs and HLA-A29 may act in concert both functionally in protecting against either infections or neoplasia and in disease pathogenesis. It may be that this combination in the past helped a portion of the population survive a bottleneck, such as the plague or other epidemic or endemic infectious disease.

The immunogenetics of KIRs suggests that this system plays additional roles in BSRC besides just explaining the favored HLA-A29/B44 haplotype. Other KIR genes found, particularly the KIR2DL/3/HLA-C1, 3DL1/Bw4 T80 and KIR2DS2/3/4 compound genotype that was found more commonly in patients with BSRC is found rarely in African Americans, another potential clue to why this disease is less common in African Americans and suggests a role for KIR bearing cells in the pathogenesis of the disease.

One hypothesis regarding the interaction of genes in the pathogenesis of BSRC is that since BSRC is found predominantly in middle aged Caucasians, despite the fact that African Americans have about half the prevalence of HLA-A29, is that immune surveillance for melanoma or other skin cancers, could play a role. This may be a good thing; we may actually find less of these cancers in patients with these genes! Of course that may be impossible to tease out as BSRC is such a rare disease and skin cancers are relatively common in Caucasians. The idea that antigens from melanoma may play a role in stimulating the immune response in HLA-A29 positive individuals was suggested by two patients reported with findings of BSRC and ocular melanoma at an American Uveitis Society meeting; the histologic findings from the eye of one of the patients has been subsequently published.[6] Of course, such melanomas are rare and this could be a chance association. While this is very speculative, it is interesting biologically and may suggest antigens to look for.

Ultimately other genes will be found to be associated with BSRC, although it is not clear whether that will impact treatment. Unlike diseases where one gene in an affected tissue plays a role, for example specific genetic defects in retinitis pigmentosa, the genetics of inflammatory, immune mediated diseases tends to be complex and genes only play a partial role in pathogenesis. Nature and nurture, including environmental factors, whether immune surveillance for cancers or infection, epigenetics or the microbiome, stress or hormones, all conspire to create a rare perfect storm like BSRC.

References

1. Zamecki KJ, Jabs DA. HLA typing in uveitis: use and misuse. *Am J Ophthalmol.* Feb 2010;149(2):189-193 e182.
2. Levinson RD, Rajalingam R, Park MS, et al. Human leukocyte antigen A29 subtypes associated with birdshot retinochoroidopathy. *Am J Ophthalmol.* Oct 2004;138(4):631-634.
3. Brezin AP, Monnet D, Cohen JH, Levinson RD. HLA-A29 and birdshot retinochoroidopathy. *Ocul Immunol Inflamm.* Dec 2011;19(6):397-400.
4. Donvito B, Monnet D, Tabary T, et al. A new HLA extended haplotype containing the A*2910 allele in birdshot retinochoroidopathy: susceptibility narrowed to the HLA molecule itself. *Invest Ophthalmol Vis Sci.* May 2010;51(5):2525-2528.
5. Levinson RD, Du Z, Luo L, et al. Combination of KIR and HLA gene variants augments the risk of developing birdshot retinochoroidopathy in HLA-A*29-positive individuals. *Genes Immun.* Apr 2008;9(3):249-258.
6. Pulido JS, Canal I, Salomao D, Kravitz D, Bradley E, Vile R. Histological findings of birdshot retinochoroidopathy in an eye with ciliochoroidal melanoma. *Eye (Lond).* Jun 2012;26(6):862-865.

Chapter 5

Outcomes with Corticosteroids

Carlos Pavesio, Bharti Arya

The management of birdshot retinochoroidopathy (BSRC) is challenging and there is currently no high level evidence to guide choice of therapeutic agent. Systemic steroids are frequently used as first line therapy in patients with BSRC and tend to have a very positive effect on retinal function and consequently on symptoms. This positive effect can be seen if they are introduced early in the course of the disease before permanent retinal damage occurs. They are usually associated with many systemic side effects making their long-term use quite problematic for most patients.

Introduction

Birdshot retinochoroidopathy (BSRC) is an uncommon condition, being diagnosed in 0.6-1.5% of patients with uveitis referred to tertiary centers, accounting for 6-7.9% of patients with posterior uveitis.[1] Females are more frequently involved and the mean age at disease onset is reported as being 53 years. The youngest reported patient was 25 years old,[2] and the oldest 79.[3]

It is found more frequently in white people of northern European origin.[4,5,6] It seems to be much less frequent in Asia, which may be related to the low prevalence of HLA-A29 among Asian populations.[1] There has been only one report of one Hispanic and one black individual with this condition.[4,7] Occurrence in families can be found, but most cases are isolated.

Clinical Manifestations

The most common symptoms related to central vision are blurring of vision and floaters, but visual acuity tends to be fairly good in the majority of patients at presentation (better than 20/40 in 61.8% of eyes),[1] despite significant complaints related to their peripheral vision. Most patients show symmetric visual acuity disturbance, but striking asymmetry can also be found. The most important reason for loss of central vision is the development of cystoid macular edema (CME). The relapsing and remitting nature of the CME may lead to permanent macular damage and permanent loss of visual acuity in later phases of the disease. Until recently, this finding represented the main reason to treat patients with BSRC, but the understanding that peripheral retinal insult is happening independent of this abnormality has led to a change in treatment strategy. The diffuse inner retinal involvement produces symptoms of reduction of peripheral visual field and nyctalopia, which are usually seen quite early, even before any other abnormalities become apparent.[8] This may be reversed by therapy and an important development in the management of BSRC has been the recognition that we should not wait for changes in central vision to initiate therapy. This is important because early and aggressive management may produce reversal of these abnormalities before they become chronic and irreversible.[9,10] It has been proposed that serial electroretinography (ERG) may be useful in monitoring response to therapy and in guiding decisions to taper medications.[9,10,11] Sequential visual field (VF) testing may also be an alternative for monitoring these patients.

Morphological and Functional Assessment

Establishing the functional status of the retina is an essential part of the therapeutic plan. Recording retinal function with the use ERG and VF provides an indication of the severity of the disease process and will allow for comparisons with the same tests carried out after therapy. The use of Spectral Domain Optical Coherence Tomography (SD-OCT) allows identification of outer retinal damage, which can also be demonstrated by fundus autofluorescence (FAF). Recent studies have indicated that it provides valuable insight into the metabolic state of the outer retina and it can demonstrate Retinal Pigment Epithelium (RPE) atrophy, which is hard to be detected by other means of investigation and do not necessarily correspond to the hypopigmented lesions clinically seen.[12,13] It may serve as a useful non-invasive assessment tool in assessing the health of the retina and potential for recovery with the presence of RPE atrophy in the macula representing an important cause of poor central visual acuity in eyes with BSCR. Fundus Fluorescein Angiography and Indocyanine Green Angiography will give an indication of the level of inflammation involving retinal vessels and the choroid respectively. These findings are also very useful in monitoring response to therapy.[14]

Therapy

BSRC is a chronic, progressive disease with the potential to cause significant visual morbidity. In order to secure the best visual outcome, the objective of therapy should be rapid achievement of maximum control of inflammatory activity followed by maintenance of control with minimum use of well tolerated agents, with the ultimate goal of maintaining remission off therapy. Systemic steroids are frequently used as first line therapy in patients with BSRC. Steroids, either systemically or locally, have also been used, especially for the treatment of CME, but also for the management of choroidal neovascular membranes (CNV), an uncommon complication in BSRC.[6,15]

Treatment with systemic steroid is likely to produce some improvement in early stages, but will not provide sufficient control. Even though long-term control may be achieved with low doses of systemic steroids, this is likely to be more an exception and they should be used more to manage acute exacerbations. There are other options including local steroids and systemic therapy with immunosuppressive agents, which are a better strategy for the long-term care of these patients.

There are no prospective studies looking at the outcomes of standalone use of systemic steroids in BSRC. A 40 year old woman experienced subjective and objective improvement following a short course of systemic corticosteroid but had an exacerbation three months after discontinuing therapy.[19] In another report, two men achieved long term control over more than four years of follow up with low dose corticosteroid and remained in remission after discontinuation of treatment.[20] In a retrospective study of 19 patients, four received Corticosteroid monotherapy. Two received treatment for intermittent exacerbations of inflammation of which in one Intermittent improvement was noted, but overall steady loss of ERG and visual field indices occurred and in the other no functional testing was performed. One patient received 6 month continuous therapy and remained stable over follow up. The fourth patient had no follow up.[21] In another retrospective study, 9 of 27 patients with five or more years of follow up received corticosteroid monotherapy. The vision improved in five eyes, remained stable in 6 eyes and deteriorated over follow up in 7 eyes. The main cause of loss of vision was cystoid macular edema.[22]

However, most of the published work is related to the use of immunosuppressive agents, many in combination, for the long term control of inflammation.[16,17,18]

The initial approach in such cases is the use of large doses of systemic steroids (prednisolone or equivalent at a dose of 1-1.5mg/kg/day) which will give an indication of the clinical response by improvement of symptoms and can be confirmed by repeat of ERG or VF carried out after initiating therapy and compared to the baseline measurements obtained before treatment. The improvement seems to correlate with angiographic reduction or resolution of retinal edema, confirmed by studies by the authors (unpublished data). This indicates that in the early stages, with significant retinal edema, it is possible to achieve a good clinical response with improvement, or even normalization, of ERG findings. In more advanced cases, when damage of the outer retina has already developed, there will be limited or no response to therapy. The ancillary tests mentioned above can already give a good indication of the likelihood of a response to therapy, but a lack of response to adequate levels of systemic steroids will confirm the irreversibility of the abnormalities. In case of a good response, the angiographic findings will show reduction of retinal vascular leakage and also of the choroidal inflammation. The functional tests should also show improvement of their findings and will be helpful in guiding treatment decisions.

Even though systemic steroids can lead to a good response with improvement of function and symptoms, they do not represent a good alternative in a chronic condition such as BSRC. The initial good response tends to regress as the level of therapy is reduced towards more acceptable levels and it is not possible in most patients to use them as single therapy. The list of side effects is quite long and for many patients they lead to a significant deterioration of their quality of life, forcing a reduction of therapy and potential deterioration of their BSRC symptoms. There are a few cases where the use of low-dose steroids (7.5mg or less of Prednisolone or equivalent) alone was sufficient to maintain long term control but these are exceptions rather than the rule.

Conclusion

Systemic steroids are a potent option that can lead to reversal of retinal dysfunction and symptoms when used in early stages of the disease but do not represent a very good alternative for maintaining control of inflammation in view of the chronic nature of the disease and the many side effects potentially associated with their long term use. They can give a good indication of the prognosis, which may justify introduction of alternative strategies with the use of immunosuppressive steroid-sparing therapy.

References

1. Shah KH, Levinson RD, Yu F, Goldhardt R, et al. Birdshot Chorioretinopathy. Surv Ophthalmol 2005 ;50 :519-41.
2. LeHoang P, Ozdemir N, Benhamou A, et al. HLA-A29.2 subtype associated with birdshot retinochoroidopathy. Am J Ophthalmol 1992;113:33-35.
3. Franceschetti A, Babel J, La chorio-retinite en "tâches de bougie," manifestation de la maladie de Besnier-Boeck. Ophthalmologica 1949 ;118 :701-710.
4. Gash At, Smith JA, Whitcupp SM. Birdshot retinochoroidopathy. Br J Ophthalmol 1999;83:241-9.
5. Gass JDM. Vitiliginous chorioretinitis. Arch Ophthalmol 1981;99:1778-1787.
6. Priem HA, Oosterhuis JA. Birdshot chrorioretinopathy : clinical characteristics and evolution. Br J Ophthalmol 1988;72:646-659.
7. Barondes MJ, Fastenberg DM, Schwartz PL, Rosen DA. Peripheral reinal neovascularization in birdshot retinochoroidopathy. Ann Ophthalmol 1989;21:306-8.
8. Soubrane G, Bokobza R, Coscas G. Late developing lesions in birdshot retinochoroidopathy. Am J Ophthalmol 1990;109:204-10.
9. Holder GE, Robson AG, Pavesio C, Graham EM. Electrophysiological characterization and monitoring in the management of birdshot chorioretinopathy. Br J Ophthalol 2005;89:709-18.
10. Sobrin L, Lam BL, Liu M et al. Electroretinographic monitoring in birdshot chorioretinopathy. Am J Ophthalmol 2005;140:52-64.

11. Zacks DN, Samson CM, Loewenstein J, Foster CS. Electroretinograms as an indicator of disease activity in birdshot retinochoroidopathy. Graefe's Arch Clin Exp Ophthalmol 2002;240:601-7.
12. Koizumi H, Pozzoni MC, Spaide RF. Fundus autofluorescence in birdshot chorioretinopathy. Ophthalmology. 2008;115:e15-20.
13. Giuliari G, Hinkle DM, Foster CS. The spectrum of fundus autofluorescence findings in birdshot chorioretinopathy. Am J Ophthalmol. 2009;2009:567-93
14. Fardeau C, Herbort CP, Kullmann N, Quentel G, LeHoang P. Indocyanine Green Angiography in birdshot chorioretinopathy. Ophthalmology. 1999 Oct;106(10):1928-34.
15. Priem HA, De Rouck A, De Laey JJ et al. Electrophysiologic studies in birdshot chorioretinopathy. Am J Ophthalmol 1988;106:430-6.
16. LeHoang P, Girard B, Deray G, et al. Cyclosporine in the treatment of birdshot retinochoroidopathy. Transplant Proc 1988;20:128-30.
17. Kiss S, Ahmed M, Letko E, Foster CS. Long-term follow-up of patients with birdshot retinochoroidopathy treated with corticosteroid-sparing systemic immunomodulatory therapy. Ophthalmology 2005;1112:1066-71.
18. Rothova A, Ossewaarde-van Norel A, Los LI, Berendschot TT. Efficacy of low-dose methotrexate treatment in birdshot chorioretinopathy. Retina. 2011 ;31:1150-5.
19. Hoffmann B . Birdshot Chorioretinopathy: Steroids and Nonsteroidal Anti-Inflammatory Drugs. Klin. Mbl. Augenheilk. 197 (1990)159-161.

20. Ladas J Arnold A, Holland G. Control of Visual Symptoms in two men with Birdshot Retinochoroidopathy Using Low- Dose Oral Corticosteroid Therapy. Am J Ophthalmol 1999;128:116–118.
21. Kean T Oh, MD[a], Nancy J Christmas, MD[a, 1], James C Folk, MD. Birdshot retinochoroiditis: long term follow-up of a chronically progressive disease. http://www.ajo.com/article/S0002-9394(02)01344-2/abstractA J Ophthalmology Volume 133, Issue 5 , Pages 622-629, May 2002.
22. H A Priem and J A Oosterhuis. Birdshot chorioretinopathy: clinical characteristics and evolution. Br J Ophthalmol1988;72:646-659 doi:10.1136/bjo.72.9.646.

Chapter 6

Outcomes with Immunomodulatory Therapy

C. Stephen Foster

Birdshot retinochoroidopathy (BSRC) results in progressive deterioration of visual function despite systemic corticosteroid therapy. Oh and associates, at the University of Iowa, may have been the first to publish data on this matter in 2002 in a paper entitled "Birdshot retinochoroidopathy: long term follow-up of a chronically progressive disease."[1] These investigators reported on 19 patients with BSRC followed for up to 220 months, with 7 of these followed for 5 years or longer. The initial visual acuity was 20/50 or better in 36 of 38 eyes and 20/60 and 20/80 in the remaining two. Visual acuity was worse than 20/50 in three of 22 eyes followed for more than 30 months. Visual field data demonstrated progressive loss of area for either the I4e or I2e isopters in six of seven patients who were followed for >or=60 months. Multiple ERGs were performed over time on eight of 19 patients; seven of eight patients demonstrated progressive loss of electrophysiologic indices. These observations led the authors to conclude that "retinal function in birdshot retinochoroidopathy deteriorated progressively over a period of years despite stable visual acuity. Late in the course of disease, visual acuity may be lost due to chorioretinal atrophy in the posterior pole. Visual acuity alone is not an adequate parameter with which to monitor disease activity and may falsely suggest that a patient is stable or doing well." The authors remarked additionally that "intermittent treatment of the inflammatory exacerbations did not prevent progressive visual loss," concluding that other treatment strategies such as immunosuppressive treatment should be investigated for patients with birdshot retinochoroidopathy.

LeHoang and colleagues had begun employing such alternative treatment, specifically cyclosporine, in their care of patients with BSRC in the 1980's, and published the results of such alternative therapy in 1988 in 21 patients, showing dramatic regression of retinal vasculitis, improved visual fields, improved electrophysiology as shown by serial electroretinography, and improved or stabilized vision in 91% of their patients.[2] The cyclosporine dose employed was 10 mg/kg or in some cases 5 mg/kg per day. The authors concluded that not only was it clear that cyclosporine was effective for the care of patients with BSRC, but also emphasized that cyclosporin "must be begun early before permanent damage."

Subsequent work with cyclosporine therapy for patients with uveitis made clear that the nephrotoxicity of the drug at the 10 mg/kg/d level was unacceptable, and so we employed a dose of 5 mg/kg/d in our patients with BSRC who had progressive loss of vision function with corticosteroid monotherapy.[3] We reported therefore, in 1994 that vitreous inflammation was controlled in 23 (88.5%) treated eyes, with fewer bouts of recurrent inflammation, and a corresponding improvement or stabilization of visual acuity in 20 (83.3%) eyes. In contrast, intraocular inflammation never was controlled fully in untreated eyes, and visual acuity decreased in six (54.5%) eyes by an average of 2.5 Snellen lines. This led us to conclude that vision preservation is possible with low-dose CSA alone or in combination with other steroid-sparing immunosuppressive agents as an alternative to the long-term use of corticosteroids, and this then became our standard of care for patients with BSRC.

In 2000, the LeHoang group from Paris reported on yet another non-steroidal therapeutic approach to the care of patients with BSRC.[4] Eighteen patients were offered therapy with infusions of intravenous immunoglobulin (IV-Ig) monthly (1.6grams/kg). The mean followup time was greater than 3 years (39 months). The authors reported that 33 of 36 eyes had improved or stable vision, and that 20 eyes demonstrated marked improvement in visual fields.

Meanwhile, other groups had begun to investigate their patients with birdshot retinochoroidopathy, all having been treated with corticosteroid monotherapy. The results were stunning. Rasquin and associates, from Belgium, reported in 2004 on patients with BSRC followed for up to 20 years.[5] They found that retinal alterations progressed despite the steroid therapy. Vision dropped, visual field and severe color vision alterations appeared and the patients complained of nyctalopia. And in that same year, Rothova and associates,[6] from The Netherlands, published a paper entitled, "Birdshot retinochoroidopathy: long-term manifestations and visual prognosis." Fifty-five patients were followed for 5 years on corticosteroid monotherapy. All patients experienced progressive deterioration of vision function. Loss of visual acuity was gradual; the number of affected eyes with visual acuity less than 20/200 increased from 9 of 108 (8%) at onset to 22 of 73 (30%) at 5 years and 19 of 49 (39%) at 10 years of follow-up, and the authors found no differences in annual loss of vision were observed between patients treated by corticosteroids and untreated patients.

And Thorne and colleagues[7] at The Johns Hopkins School of Medicine similarly analyzed their cohort of patients with BSRC, finding that patients who presented with a duration of disease of two and a half or more years had higher frequencies of visual impairment to 20/50 or worse (68% vs 32%) and to 20/200 or worse (32% vs 9%) compared to patients who presented with a duration of disease less than 30 months . The incidence rates on follow-up for vision loss to 20/50 or worse and to 20/200 or worse were 13% and 4% per eye-year (EY), respectively. The authors concluded that "use of immunosuppressive drug therapy was associated with a reduced risk of vision loss."

The Foster group published a long term followup report of twenty-eight patients with a mean follow-up of 81.2 months.[8] None had control of their inflammation before referral. All patients were treated with corticosteroid-sparing systemic immunomodulatory therapy; 92.9% were treated with cyclosporine, 67.9% with mycophenolate mofetil, 17.9% with azathioprine, 10.7% with oral methotrexate, and 7.1% with daclizumab. Average Snellen visual acuities at the time of initial visit were 0.64 (right eye) and 0.59 (left eye). Average final Snellen visual acuities were 0.74 (right eye) and 0.71 (left eye), i.e., improved vision. Visual fields also improved, and electrophysiology either improved or did not continue to deteriorate. This led us to conclude "Long-term preservation of visual function is attainable with systemic corticosteroid-sparing immunomodulatory therapy (IMT) for patients with BSRC. Prompt treatment with systemic IMT may offer the best hope of maintaining retinal function in what is often thought of as a chronically progressive disease resistant to treatment."

Rothova's study of 147 eyes in 76 patients is the largest series published to date.[9] Seventy-eight eyes were in patients with no therapy; 37 eyes were in patients with corticosteroid therapy; and 32 eyes were in patients with methotrexate therapy. The authors reported that the visual acuity at initial visit strongly correlated with final vision, with loss of visual acuity and of visual field most prominent in the corticosteroid and no therapy groups. All eyes deteriorating to the level of legal blindness were in patients who had had no drug therapy or in the corticosteroid treated groups. The eyes of patients treated with methotrexate fared better than the eyes of patients in the other groups. And the data indicated that early therapy with methotrexate was clearly superior in outcomes to therapy with corticosteroid monotherapy.

Finally, the Foster group at the Massachusetts Eye Research and Surgery Institution (MERSI) in Cambridge, Massachusetts reported on the one year outcomes of 49 patients with BSRC treated with combination mycophenolate mofetil and cyclosporine.[10] Vitreous inflammation was significantly reduced from baseline in all patients; retinal vasculitis was significantly reduced from baseline; the 30

Hz implicit times were significantly improved from baseline on Ganzfeld ERG assessments every 6 months, and vision was preserved in every patient. The median duration of disease was 65 months, and the median duration of therapy was 17 months. Thus, there was a very substantial delay in referral to MERSI for immunomodulatory therapy.

I believe that the matter of proper care of patients with birdshot retinochoroidopathy is a settled matter. Corticosteroid therapy is not appropriate. Immunomodulatory therapy is clearly the standard of care, with clear evidence that such therapy preserves vision and visual function in most patients so treated. It is not clear if one immunomodulatory approach is superior to another, but it is quite clear that the patient with BSRC should be educated about the evidence in peer reviewed literature on this matter of corticosteroid therapy versus immunodulatory therapy.

References

1. Oh, K. T., Christmas, N. J. & Folk, J. C. Birdshot retinochoroiditis: long term follow-up of a chronically progressive disease. *Am. J. Ophthalmol.* **133,** 622–629 (2002).
2. Le Hoang, P. *et al.* Cyclosporine in the treatment of birdshot retinochoroidopathy. *Transplant. Proc.* **20,** 128–130 (1988).
3. Vitale, A. T., Rodriguez, A. & Foster, C. S. Low-dose cyclosporine therapy in the treatment of birdshot retinochoroidopathy. *Ophthalmology* **101,** 822–831 (1994).
4. LeHoang, P., Cassoux, N., George, F., Kullmann, N. & Kazatchkine, M. D. Intravenous immunoglobulin (IVIg) for the treatment of birdshot retinochoroidopathy. *Ocul. Immunol. Inflamm.* **8,** 49–57 (2000).
5. Rasquin, F. A. & Pereleux, A. A. Long term follow-up of birdshot chorioretinopathy. *Bull. Société Belge Ophtalmol.* 25–33 (2004).
6. Rothova, A., Berendschot, T. T. J. M., Probst, K., van Kooij, B. & Baarsma, G. S. Birdshot chorioretinopathy: long-term manifestations and visual prognosis. *Ophthalmology* **111,** 954–959 (2004).
7. Thorne, J. E. *et al.* Birdshot retinochoroidopathy: ocular complications and visual impairment. *Am. J. Ophthalmol.* **140,** 45–51 (2005).
8. Kiss, S., Ahmed, M., Letko, E. & Foster, C. S. Long-term follow-up of patients with birdshot retinochoroidopathy treated with corticosteroid-sparing systemic immunomodulatory therapy. *Ophthalmology* **112,** 1066–1071 (2005).
9. Rothova, A., Ossewaarde-van Norel, A., Los, L. I. & Berendschot, T. T. J. M. Efficacy of low-dose methotrexate treatment in birdshot chorioretinopathy. *Retina Phila. Pa* **31,** 1150–1155 (2011).
10. Cervantes-Castañeda, R. A., Gonzalez-Gonzalez, L. A., Cordero-Coma, M., Yilmaz, T. & Foster, C. S. Combined therapy of cyclosporine A and mycophenolate mofetil for the treatment of birdshot retinochoroidopathy: a 12-month follow-up. *Br. J. Ophthalmol.* **97,** 637–643 (2013).

Chapter 7

Best Monitoring Practices

Henry J. Kaplan, Niloofar Piri

Birdshot retinochoroidopathy (BSRC) is a disease that requires very careful objective monitoring. Patients with this disease may retain very good central visual acuity and have few subjective complaints, but the disease, particularly the outer retinopathy, can progress and result in significant loss of dark adaptation and peripheral visual field. Fortunately, we now have several objective tests that can be routinely performed so that immunosuppressive or immunomodulatory therapy can be implemented as required.

Birdshot retinochoroidopathy (BSRC) is a chronic, progressive disease with complications including vitritis, cystoid macular edema (CME), retinal vasculitis, and progressive photoreceptor cell death. Although the etiology of the disease is unknown, it appears to be immune mediated – most likely involving both autoinflammation and autoimmunity. The clinical manifestations of the disease, both subjective and objective, are a reflection of both inner and outer retinopathy. Close monitoring of objective visual function in these patients is critical to prevent slowly progressive, irreversible visual loss from outer retinal damage. The clinical monitoring of patients with BSRC requires both subjective and objective testing. We will review the role of all of these tests and conclude with our personal routine at the University of Louisville in the monitoring of patients with this disease.

Visual Acuity

Visual acuity alone is not an adequate parameter with which to monitor disease activity and may falsely suggest that a patient is stable or doing well.[1] In many patients there is loss of retinal function documented by progressive deterioration of visual fields over a period of years despite stable visual acuity. Although symptoms may be present in patients with BSRC, even among those with good best corrected visual acuity, no relationship between birdshot lesion characteristics and visual acuity has been demonstrated.[2] These findings highlight the limitation of using visual acuity for clinical monitoring of patients with BSRC, as well as an outcome measure for studies of this disease.

Imaging

Color fundus images are helpful to document the presence of BSRC lesions but are not useful to monitor progression of the disease. Even fluorescein angiography (FA) has limited usefulness, being most frequently used to confirm the presence of CME, retinal vasculitis (in medium-sized and capillary retinal vessels) and optic disc edema.[3] Herbort and colleagues noticed a pseudo-perfusion delay in the FA of BSRC with incomplete filling of large veins, in contrast to indocyanine green angiography (ICGA) which showed complete arterio-venous filling without delay. In addition, on ICGA they observed hypofluorescent dark dots (HDDs) in the choroid and fuzzy choroidal vessels in both symptomatic and asymptomatic eyes.

Ocular coherence tomography (OCT) imaging, particularly spectral domain OCT (SD-OCT), are among the useful objective studies to monitor patients with BSRC. Monnet et al[4] noticed that symptoms were most closely related to loss of the third hyperreflective band in BSRC patients. Additionally, systemic immunosuppression has been documented on OCT to result in the restoration of retinal architecture. OCT is most helpful in documenting the presence of CME (i.e. intraretinal fluid accumulation caused by capillary leakage from the parafoveal retinal vasculature), as well as diffuse macular edema from compromise of the tight junctions in the retinal pigment epithelium. Most recently, the use of enhanced depth OCT imaging has revealed retinal changes outside the macula including patchy disruption of the photoreceptor IS/OS junction (i.e. the ellipsoid layer), generalized thinning of the retina, and patchy disruption of the RPE.[6] Patches of small hyperreflective foci were also seen with disruption of the photoreceptor IS/OS junction. These lesions may represent clumping of the photoreceptors in response to injury or areas of intraretinal pigment migration.

Electrophysiology

Electrophysiologic studies demonstrate early loss of oscillatory potentials and b-wave amplitudes as a consequence of the inner retinopathy in BSRC. Later in the course of the disease, the photopic b-wave amplitude and flicker response are decreased reflecting impaired outer retinal function as the result of outer retinopathy. Foster's group[7] observed that the ERG can predict success in tapering of immunosuppressive medication in patients with BSRC. Although seven parameters of the ERG were examined in patients with recurrent intraocular inflammation only abnormalities in the bright scotopic response amplitudes and the 30 Hz flicker implicit times were associated with recurrence as immunosuppressive therapy was tapered. Indeed, the most sensitive parameter for retinal dysfunction is the delayed implicit time in the 30 Hz cone flicker response,[8,9] which was most often associated with other clinically important parameters such as duration of symptoms and deviation from normal. Holder et al[8] also noted a significant improvement in retinal function following immunosuppressive therapy. This observation led to the recommended treatment strategy in which ERG data are used to decide when to start treatment in BSRC and when to reinstitute treatment after it is tapered. Holder confirmed that clinical features were not reliable indicators of functional deterioration or recovery. Only objective electrophysiological assessment of retinal function was associated with improvement following treatment and provided a reliable method of monitoring treatment efficacy. The importance of the 30 Hz implicit time was also noted by Comander et al.[10] They observed that a normal implicit time was the most reliable correlation with successful taper from systemic immunomodulatory therapy without recurrence.

Visual Fields

A variety of visual field abnormalities was seen even in patients with normal best corrected visual acuity. The mean deviation was the parameter in automated visual field testing most commonly related to clinical disease activity and is important in clinical care, as well as research.[11] Thorne et al.[12] observed that Goldmann visual field testing was more sensitive in detecting visual field loss than mean deviation from the Humphrey automated perimeter. Of the 36 eyes in which the I-4 isopter was abnormal on Goldmann visual field and in which Humphrey fields were also available, only five eyes (14%) were also abnormal on Humphrey visual field testing. However, the reliability and reproducibility of the Goldmann visual field is examiner dependent, so that other tests such as the ERG are more reliable in documenting a change in retinal function. Although an abnormal visual field may improve with immunomodulatory therapy, when eyes with inactive BSRC were compared with control eyes there was a statistically significant difference in threshold sensitivity $\leq$16dB, suggesting that not all patients recover their full retinal sensitivity.[13] These observations suggest that the quality of vision is not reflective of visual acuity measured with standard testing.

Color Vision and Contrast Sensitivity

Color vision can be abnormal in eyes with normal visual acuity.[14] Color vision testing with the desaturated Lanthony 15-Hue test was abnormal in almost half of patients with BSRC. Therefore, this test may be useful as an additional measure for monitoring disease progression. Similarly, decreased contrast sensitivity is common in patients with BSRC and may occur in the absence of other visual changes.[15] Therefore, contrast sensitivity may also be useful for clinical studies of BSRC and for monitoring patients with the disease.

Our Approach at the University of Louisville

We obtain baseline studies on all patients diagnosed with BSRC. Specifically, we obtain color fundus images, FA and ICGA, enhanced depth imaging with SD-OCT, automated Humphrey visual field 30-2, dark adaptation, full field ERG and multifocal ERG. Every six months we repeat the enhanced SD-OCT (to detect CME, epiretinal membrane formation, and/or alteration in retinal structure), Humphrey visual field 30-2, dark adaptation and full field ERG regardless of clinical appearance. A FA and ICGA are repeated for patient complaints or if the visual acuity is decreased and clinical examination or other tests are not revealing.

In conclusion, BSRC is a disease that can progress inexorably with minimal subjective clinical complaints. Therefore, it is important to monitor BSRC patients with objective tests to determine if immunomodulatory therapy needs to be implemented or to determine if such therapy can be tapered.

References

1. Oh KT, Christmas NJ, Folk JC. Birdshot retinochoroidopathy: long term follow-up of a chronically progressive disease. Am J Ophthalmol. 2002:133(5):622-9.
2. Monnet J, Brezin AP, Holland GN, et al. Longitudinal cohort study of patients with birdshot retinochoroidopathy. I. Baseline clinical characteristics. Am J Ophthalmol. 2006:141(1):135-42.
3. Papadia M, Herbort CP. Reappraisal of birdshot retinochoroidopathy (BSRC): a global approach. Graefes Arch Clin Exp Ophthalmol. 2013:251(3):861-9.
4. Monnet D, Levinson RD, Holland GN, et al. Longitudinal cohort study of patients with birdshot retinochoroidopathy. III. Macular imaging at baseline. Am J Ophthalmol. 2007:144(6):818-28.
5. Forooghian F, Gulati N, Jabs DA. Restoration of retinal architecture following systemic immunosuppression in birdshot retinochoroidopathy. Ocul Immunol Inflamm. 2010:18(6):470-1.
6. Keane PA, MRCOpth, MSc, et al. When you can have the bird without shooting it!: extramacular enhanced depth optical coherence tomography in birdshot retinochoroidopathy. JAMA Ophthalmol. 2013:131(10):1369-70.
7. Zacks DN, Samson CM, Loewenstein J, et al. Electroretinograms as an indicator of disease activity in birdshot retinochoroidopathy. Graefes Arch Clin Exp Ophthalmol. 2002:240(8):601-7.
8. Holder GE, Robson AG, Pavesio C, et al. Electrophysiological characterization and monitoring in the management of birdshot retinochoroidopathy. Br J Ophthalmol. 2005:89(6):709-18.

9. Sorbin L, Lam BL, Liu M, et al. Electroretinographic monitoring in birdshot retinochoroidopathy. Am J. Ophthalmol. 2005:140(1):52-64.
10. Comander J, Loewenstein J, Sorbin L: Diagnostic testing and monitoring in birdshot retinochoroidopathy. Semin Ophthalmol. 2011:26(4-5):329-36.
11. Gordon LK, Monnet D, Holland GN, et al. Longitudinal cohort study of patients with birdshot retinochoroidopathy. IV. Visual field results at baseline. Am J Ophthalmol. 2007:144(6):829-37.
12. Thorne JE, Jabs DA, Kedhar SR, et al. Loss of visual field among patients with birdshot retinochoroidopathy. Am J Ophthalmol. 2008:145(1):23-28.
13. Giuliari GP, Pujari S, Shaikh M, et al. Microperimetry findings in patients with birdshot retinochoroidopathy. Can J Ophthalmol. 2010:45(4):399-403.
14. Holland GN, Shah KH, Monnet D. Longitudinal cohort study of patients with birdshot retinochoroidopathy II: color vision at baseline. Am J Ophthalmol. 2006:142(6):1013-8.
15. Kappel PJ, Monnet D, Yu F, et al. Contrast sensitivity among patients with birdshot retinochoroidopathy. Am J Ophthalmol. 2009:147(2):351-56.

Chapter 8

Rectifications in the Appraisal of BSRC

Carl P. Herbort Jr., Marina Papadia

The first reports on birdshot retinochoroidopathy (BSRC) date back just over 30 years. This posterior uveitis with dual, independent retinal and choroidal inflammation is a puzzling disease, and various misconceptions and omissions have hampered its correct appraisal. The disease has no known extraocular inflammation sites and yet features the strongest known HLA association: HLA-A29 is present in close to 100% of cases. Initial reports described BSRC in detail, employing precise observation and investigational procedures available at that time. Some of the clinical features described (e.g., the presence of keratic precipitates) were not mentioned in subsequent reports, likely because the series reported were usually small. Retinal involvement was clearly characterized, pointing out the profuse leakage of retinal vessels of all sizes in early disease. Initial reports on inefficacy of corticosteroids together with the erroneous use of visual acuity rather than visual field testing to make treatment decisions led to insufficient therapy for decades. Exploration of the choroid was unavailable until the early 1990s before the advent of indocyanine green angiography (ICGA). Despite its proven importance to explore the choroid, ICGA is still sparsely used. The diagnostic criteria that were generated based on these misconceptions are inappropriate and do not allow early diagnosis.

The aim of this work was to point out incongruities, omissions and misconceptions in the clinical approach to birdshot retinochoroidopathy (BSRC) since its initial description in 1980–1981. We give our appraisal of the disease, taking into account all investigational procedures at our disposal to foster a global, comprehensive and precise approach to BSRC.

This is not an exhaustive review; points will mainly be addressed at which our approach has diverged from common practice during the last 33 years. These points include historical background; nomenclature; disease description and disease mechanism; diagnostic investigations and functional testing including fundus photography, fluorescein angiography (FA), indocyanine green angiography (ICGA), optical coherence tomography (OCT), visual field testing, electrophysiology and HLA typing; diagnostic criteria; and treatment and evolution. Discrepancies versus the commonly used approach will be highlighted.

Historical Background

Birdshot retinochoroidopathy is a rare, bilateral, retinochoroidal, inflammatory disease without known systemic involvement; it is mostly seen in Caucasians.[1] It is a relatively recently recognized entity, as it was first described in 1980 by Ryan and Maumenee.[2] In 1981, Gass described 11 similar cases and called the disease vitiliginous chorioretinitis.[3] Like Ryan and Maumenee, he described keratic precipitates (KPs) in two patients and mutton-fat precipitates on the posterior surface of the detached vitreous in two additional patients. This fact was never mentioned in subsequent series and became an exclusion criterion in the research diagnostic criteria decided upon in a consensus workshop on BSRC held in 2002 and published in 2006.[4] An important FA sign that Gass observed was the loss of fluorescein into the retina and the weak fluorescein coloration of large veins, which indicated an increased delay in retinal circulation, a finding that we have been able to explain using dual FA/ICGA (see below).[5] He correctly attributed the depigmented areas to the loss of choroidal stromal melanocytes. He also contributed to the belief that corticosteroids were of little efficacy. The next milestone article, which was published by Nussenblatt et al. in 1982, associated HLA-A29 antigen with the disease.[6] Another crucial article in the appraisal of BSRC by Gaudio et al. provided a histopathological description of birdshot lesions, showing that there were infiltrates around the choroidal stromal melanocytes; they were of partial thickness; did not touch the choriocapillaris/retinal pigment epithelium complex or the sclera; and had granulomatous features.[7]

Nomenclature

In the first article on the disease, Ryan and Maumenee chose the name of birdshot retinochoroidopathy, placing "retino-" before "choroid".[2] In his article, Gass chose to call the disease vitiliginous chorioretinitis placing "choroid" first.[3] In both articles, the choroidal involvement was at the origin of the first term of the eponym as both "birdshot" and "vitiliginous" refer to the rice-shaped, depigmented choroidal fundus lesions that characterize the condition. Of the two denominations, there is no question that "birdshot" is the universally used and accepted term. It is unfortunate that the condition was called a retinochoroidopathy in the first published article, although the authors clearly acknowledged its inflammatory character.[2] The inflammatory character appears more clearly in the name chosen by Gass, as he speaks of vitiliginous chorioretin*itis*. It is now clear that BSRC is not a retinochoroido*pathy*; the suffix "pathy" indicates a non-inflammatory condition, as is the case for central serous chorioretinopathy. As the nature of the condition is clearly inflammatory, obviously the suffix "itis" should be used. The last question regarding the denomination is the choice of the second term of the eponym. Should "retino-" precede "choroid" or vice versa, a point on which the two initial articles were contradictory.[2,3] In full-blown or late disease, the clinical signs that strike the clinician most are the depigmented lesions that led to the terms "vitiliginous" and "birdshot". This clearly observable characteristic also influenced some authors to give precedence to the choroid over the retina in the second term of the eponym, speaking of chorioretinitis. It is our opinion that attention should be given to the early phase of the disease, referred to as the exudative phase of BSRC. During this phase, retinal involvement is preponderant over the choroidal lesions, which remain occult and are only detectable using ICGA. Additionally, the retina is the structure from which most of the disease morbidity originates. For both of these reasons the disease should be called "birdshot retinochroiditis" rather than the other way around.

DISEASE DESCRIPTION & MECHANISM

Disease Characteristics

Birdshot retinochoroidopathy is an intraocular inflammatory condition without any known systemic associations. It involves both the retina and the choroid and is linked in nearly all cases to the presence of the HLA-A29 human leucocyte histocompatibility antigen. The disease occurs almost exclusively in Caucasians and affects patients in their 50s, with a female:male ratio of 1.5:1.

Anterior Segment Inflammation: BSRC Is a Granulomatous Uveitis

Anterior segment inflammation is mild to subclincal and frank anterior chamber inflammation is rare. In a collective of 13 patients (26 eyes) where measurements were available at presentation, laser flare photometry revealed a mean flare value of 10.6 ph/ms in treatment-naïve patients.[8] This finding indicates that there is minimal anterior spillover inflammation in this posterior uveitis and therefore laser flare photometry is not suitable for monitoring disease activity in most cases.[9] However, since the early reports by both Ryan and Maumenee and Gass, KPs were no longer described, even leading a group of experts to list the presence of KPs as an exclusion criterion.[4] We found small granulomatous KPs in 3/19 (16%) treatment-naïve BSRC patients (Figure 1).[10]patients (Figure 1).[10] One single granulomatous KP was detected in two of these patients, a feature also described by Gass in his first report. This very discrete occurrence of KPs might be the reason why in subsequent reports the presence of KPs was overlooked; a series of at least 8-9 treatment-naïve patients is needed to have one case that may show only one KP. It is therefore puzzling that the presence of KPs was not mentioned in a study of 80 BSRC patients examined at baseline.[11]

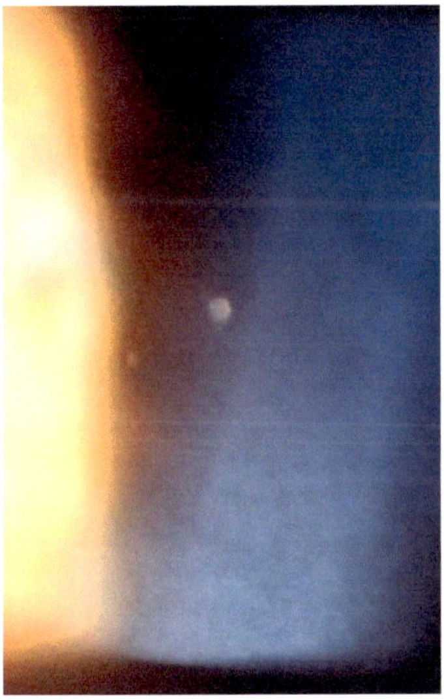

Figure 1. Granulomatous keratic precipitates (KPs) in a treatment-naïve patient. Disease had been evolving without treatment for 10 years when this single granulomatous KP was observed. A second smaller KP is visible to the left of the medium-sized KP.

Vitritis

All reports indicate unanimously that inflammation in this compartment always shows cells, giving the fuzzy fundus observed in most treatment-naïve patients. Vitritis is a constant feature in BSRC. Ryan and Maumenee describe debris and opacities in all of their patients, however Gass clearly described cells in all 11 of his patients, of which one had 1+ cells, six had 2+ cells and four had 3+ cells. In two cases he described "mutton-fat precipitates on the posterior surface of the detached vitreous humor".

Retinal Involvement

Retinal signs observed on fundus examination can include retinal vasculitis of large veins and papillitis, but retinal disease is most clearly demonstrated by FA. Patients usually present with vitreous symptoms that include floaters and fuzzy vision, as well as retinal symptoms such as dimness of vision, fluctuating vision, subjective scotomas and peripheral vision difficulties. In the presence of vitritis, these symptoms lead the clinician to perform FA and OCT, which best illustrate retinal involvement (see below).

Choroidal Involvement

Rice-shaped depigmented BSRC fundus lesions were the hallmark sign that allowed the identification and discovery of this entity and turned out to be one of the main disease-defining criteria (Figure 2). It was not possible to explore choroidal involvement in more detail at the time when the disease was initially described, as ICGA became available only in the early 1990s.[12,13] Today, after the advent of ICGA and the histopathological findings reported by Gaudio et al.,[7] it is clear that choroidal inflammation in BSRC belongs to the category of primary stromal choroiditis, which also in-

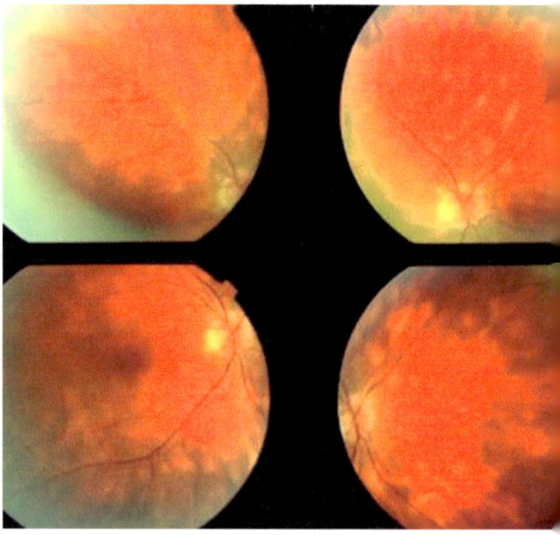

Figure 2. Typical depigmented rice-shaped birdshot lesions (BSRC fundus lesions) in a patient that declined treatment for 10 years.

cludes Vogt-Koyanagi-Harada (VKH) disease and sympathetic ophthalmia. Unlike these two latter conditions (which are purely primary stromal choroiditis), BSRC is indeed a primary stromal choroiditis, but not only, as additional unrelated retinitis is also present. Choroidal ICGA lesions appear very early in the disease, but remain occult unless ICGA is performed or until BSRC fundus lesions. Choroidal involvement is best demonstrated by ICGA (see below).

Disease Mechanisms

In his report, Gass found many similarities between BSRC and VKH disease and his comparisons were highly pertinent. The choroidal stroma is the site of inflammation in both diseases and stromal melanocytes are the target of the immune reaction. The immune reaction leads to depigmentation, which takes on the aspect of sunset glow fundus in VKH and the aspect of rice-shaped depigmented BSRC fundus lesions in BSRC. Choroidal inflammation is characterized by primary stromal choroiditis in both diseases, meaning that the primary obligatory site of inflammation is located in the choroidal stroma.[14] The antigen that triggers the immune reaction to cause inflammation in the choroidal stroma has been determined in VKH, but is unknown in BSRC.[15]

There are other significant differences between these two stromal choroiditis entities. The primary inflammatory process in VKH is limited to the choroidal stroma. It is a much more severe choroiditis that fills out the entire thickness of the choroid and causes significant secondary inflammation in neighboring structures such as the retina, vitreous compartment and optic nerve head; this is the stage when the disease becomes clinically apparent.[16] BSRC is a stromal choroiditis, but not only, as inflammatory events involve both the retina and the choroid in parallel and independently. Also, unlike in VKH, retinal inflammation in BSRC is not the consequence of choroiditis. This is also the reason why aggressive treatment of VKH rapidly resolves inflammation in both compartments (which is not the case in BSRC, in which retinal inflammation is more resistant because it is autonomous and not caused by spillover choroidal inflammation). Because of this dual independent parallel inflammation, the choroidal response to treatment (as judged by the resolution of ICGA signs) was rapid and complete, while the response of retinal disease was much less satisfactory (Figure 3).[17]

BSRC should undoubtedly be classified as a granulomatous uveitis. This assessment is based clinically on the granolumatous KPs observed in 15% to 20% of cases and the mutton-fat precipitates on the detached posterior vitreous described by Gass. The histopathology report by Gaudio et al. also described granulomatous features in the infiltrates around the islets of stromal melanocytes.

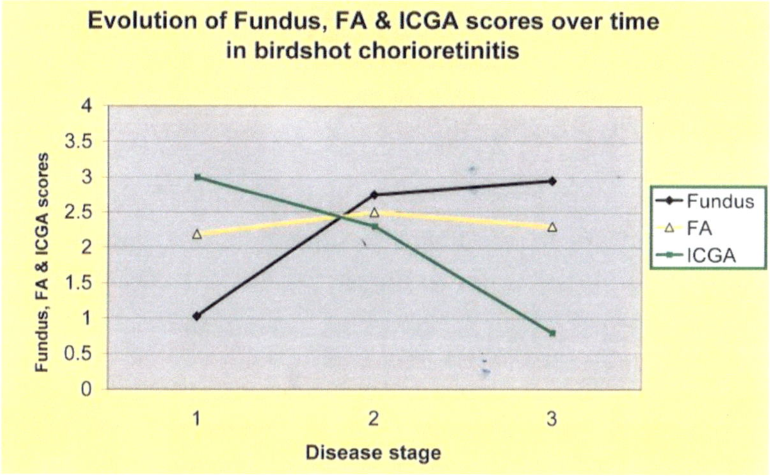

Figure 3. Differential response to the treatment of retinal and choroidal inflammation. At presentation (stage 1), occult disease is maximal, but responds satisfactorily to treatment (measured by ICGA; green line). The mean BSRC fundus score at presentation shows that when BSRC fundus lesions are already present at treatment initiation, they tend to increase despite treatment until late stage (>7 years of disease progression; black line). Retinal disease is stabilized (yellow line). (from Klin Monbl Augenheilkd, 2004; 221:351-6)

The natural history of BSRC is classically divided into an early stage and a late stage of disease. During the early stage, called the exudative stage, diffuse leakage from small and large retinal vessels causes diffuse retinal edema on FA and thickening on OCT. BSRC fundus lesions may not yet be visible during this stage. During the later disease stages, choroidal BSRC fundus lesions appear progressively and the retina evolves towards atrophy and thinning with thinned retinal vessels representing the atrophic stage of the disease.This evolution can be avoided to some extent if treatment is started early.

DIAGNOSTIC INVESTIGATIONS & FUNCTIONAL TESTING

Fundus Photography

Fundus photography is useful for following BSRC fundus lesions and allows clinicians to document changes that occur between visits (refer to Figure 2).

Fluorescein Angiography

Fluorescein angiography (FA) is routinely performed in patients that present with the above-mentioned symptoms that are compatible with BSRC and associated with vitritis. In the absence of any additional investigation (such as ICGA), the condition is often misdiagnosed as retinal vasculitis. Retinal inflammatory involvement in BSRC is best diagnosed using FA.

During the early exudative stage of BSRC there are at least three characteristic signs that are observable using FA. In the early angiographic frames Gass (very accurately) observed "an increased retinal circulation delay". He also perspicaciously noted that in all patients "there was a varying degree of unexplained subnormal fluorescence of the retinal vessels during the entire course of the angiography".[3] By performing dual FA/ICGA we showed that retinal circulation time is actually not increased; early ICGA frames show that large veins are marked by ICG within a normal time interval.[5] This FA pseudo-delay is explained by the diffuse capillary exudation of fluorescein to the extent that there is not enough dye to normally mark the large veins. In contrast, the large ICG complex does not leak from retinal capillaries and normally marks large veins, which indicates that there is no real hemodynamic slowing (Figure 4). Consequently, the first specific FA sign in BSRC is massive and diffuse retinal capillary leakage with diffuse retinal edema, which was also described by Gass (Figure 5).

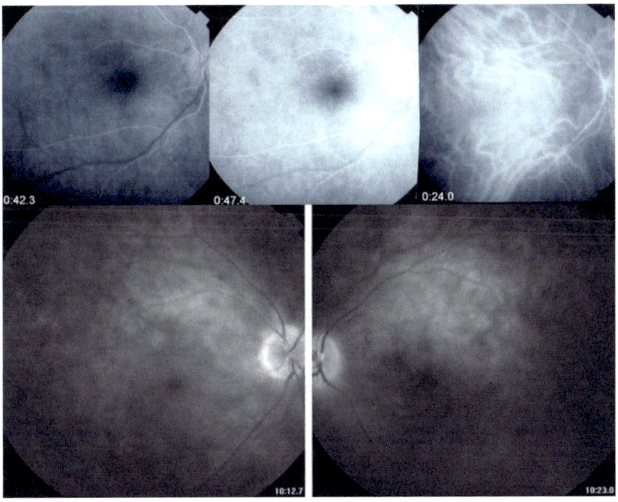

Figure 4. Pseudo-delay in retinal circulation. A patient in the exudative stage of BSRC exhibits no fluorescein marking of large veins at 42.3 s. (top left) and 47.4 s (top middle) after injection. This is not due to an increase of arterio-venous circulation time, but to massive extrusion of the small fluorescein molecule from retinal capillaries and larger vessels. This phenomenon is revealed by ICGA; opacification of large veins occurs normally at 24.0 s (top right), as the large ICG complex does not extrude from retinal vessels. Late FA frames from the same patient reveal massive and diffuse retinal edema, which explains the massive loss of fluorescein . Note that despite diffuse edema, the fovea remains relatively spared, which allows 20/20 bilateral vision.

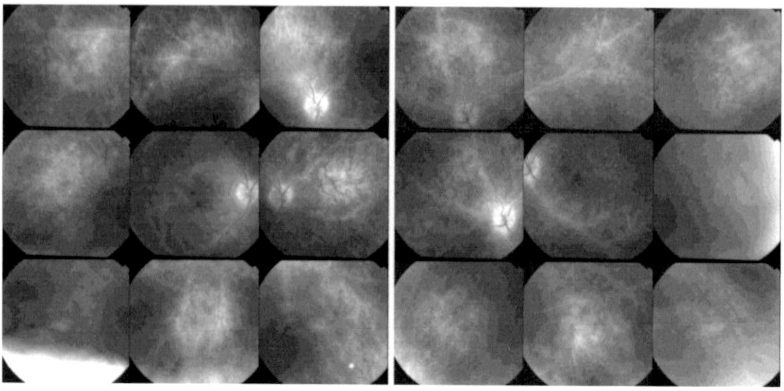

Figure 5. Profuse retinal vasculitis and disc hyperfluorescence. A patient in the exudative stage of BSRC (the same patient as in Figure 4) exhibits extensive vasculitis of small vessels and large veins (caused by retinal inflammation) accounting for the patient's visual field impairment.

This diffuse retinal edema also involves the macula, but strangely the foveal area appears to be spared often, which explains the good vision retained by a large proportion of patients for a relatively long period of time. In a recent study we showed that true cystoid macular edema was not as frequent as indicated in the literature and that the central fovea might be devoid of leakage, even in cases with diffuse retinal and macular edema (Figure 6).[18] Although veins are often barely visible in early frames, in later frames there is leakage along large veins. This later leakage often leads to the erroneous diagnosis of retinal vasculitis if ICGA is not performed, and this represents the second significant FA sign in BSRC (Figure 5). The third sign is disc hyperfluorescence, which is almost always present (Figure 5).

At a later stage of BSRC, FA shows diffuse thinning of vessels including arteries and veins. Such thinning is a consequence of an extensive atrophic retinal process, which can be partially avoided by early and sustained IST management.

Optical Coherence Tomography

Optical coherence tomography (OCT) allows another approach and provides a morphological explanation for the retinal signs observed using FA. We showed that in early disease a diffusely thickened retina was measured in the macula, but less so in the fovea, which exhibited fewer fluctuations in thickness during disease progression. This supports the FA finding showing that the fovea was relatively spared.[19] After a few years of disease progression, OCT revealed both areas of atrophy/thinning and areas of thickening, while in late disease the mean retinal thickness was reduced (mostly in patients for which treatment had been delayed) (Figure 7). Optical coherence tomography also provided information about the vitreo-retinal interface; it revealed the presence of thin, pauci-contractile epiretinal membranes in up to 93% of cases.[19]

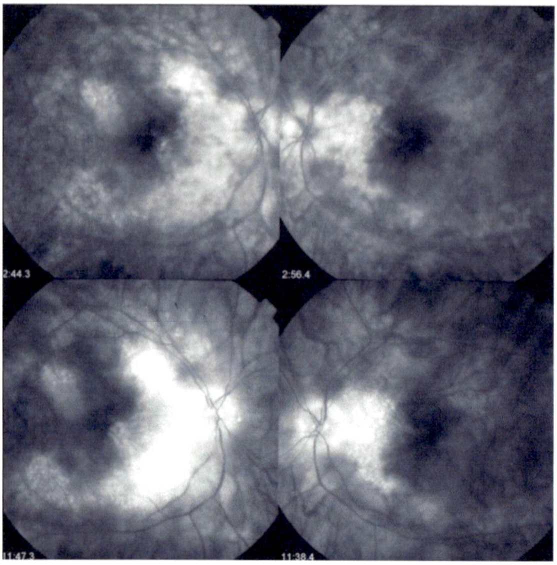

Figure 6. Foveal sparing of diffuse retinal edema. This patient was followed for more than 7 years for "neuroretinitis", without treatment. ICGA revealed numerous hypofluorescent dark dots bilaterally (not shown). There is massive retinal edema that also involves the posterior pole, yet the fovea remains relatively spared, which explains the patient's preserved visual acuity.

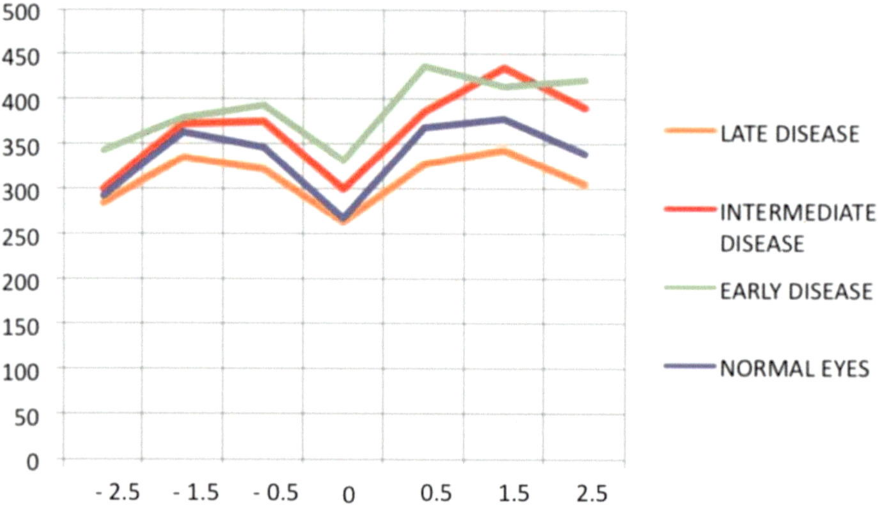

Figure 7. Progression of retinal disease as followed by optical coherence tomography (x axis indicates distance from fovea (=0); y axis indicates thickness of retina in microns). Early disease (green line) features thickening of the retina (and to a lesser degree the fovea). In late disease (yellow line) there is diffuse thinning except in the fovea; foveal thickness remains comparable to normals (purple line) (from Ophthalmic Surg Lasers Imaging 2012; 43-suppl S25-31).

Indocyanine Green Angiography Is an Essential Tool for Early Diagnosis

Indocyanine green angiography (ICGA) became available for clinical use in the early 1990s and enabled insight into choroidal inflammation.[20] One substantial advantage of this method is that it made possible the detection of occult choroidal lesions that were inaccessible when other investigational methods were used. Despite this undisputed advantage, many centers still do not use ICGA routinely.[21] ICGA allows clinicians to subdivide choroidal inflammation into choriocapillaritis entities (e.g., multiple evanescent white dot syndrome or acute posterior multifocal placoid pigment epitheliopathy) on one side and stromal choroiditis (e.g., VKH and BSRC) on the other.[22] Despite its obvious advantage to the investigation of choroiditis, publications on ICGA in BSRC are scarce. To date, of the 240 articles on BSRC listed in PubMed, fewer than 10 publications have a strong focus on ICGA. We standardized ICGA findings in BSRC in 1999[23] and in 2011 we showed that ICGA is essential to establish an early diagnosis of BSRC.[24]

Relevant ICGA signs for diagnosis and disease monitoring are the presence of hypofluorescent dark dots (HDDs) and fuzziness of large choroidal vessels (Figure 8). HDDs were suspected to be caused by stromal inflammatory foci; this hypothesis was confirmed histologically by Gaudio et al.[7] Many HDDs become isofluorescent on late angiographic frames, which indicates that (unlike in VKH) lesions do not occupy the full thickness of the choroidal stroma; this

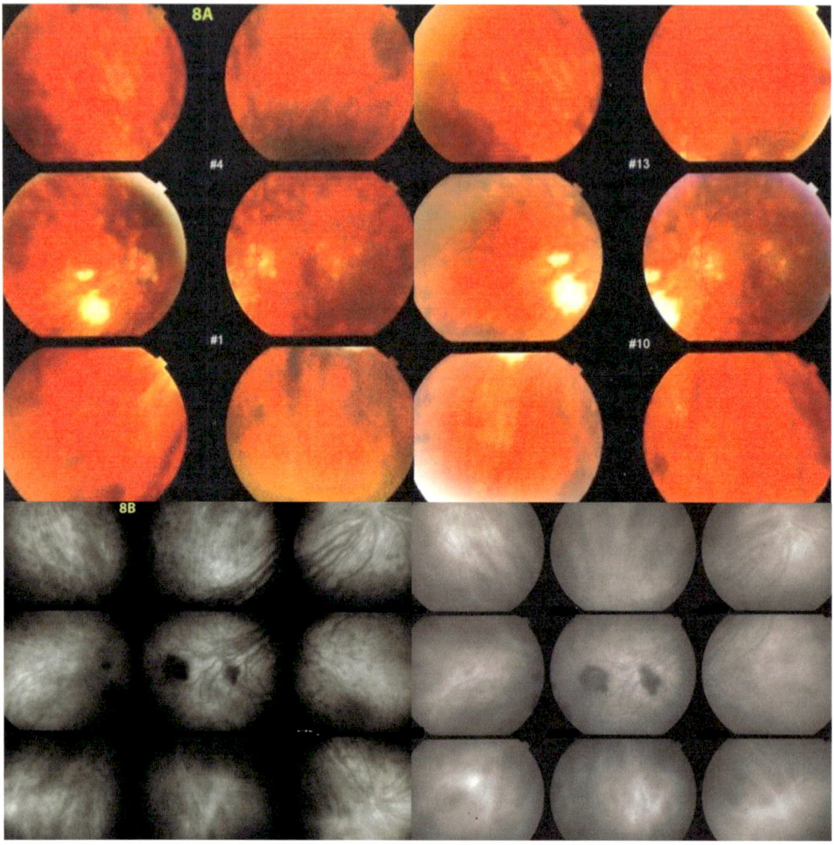

Figure 8. Indocyanine green angiography (ICGA) lesions do not correspond to birdshot retinochoroidopathy (BSRC) fundus lesions. This woman was 64 years old at presentation; her history featured a 32-month diagnostic delay and a 38-month treatment delay (left eye). Fundus images before treatment (A, left sextet of images) reveal well-delineated BSRC fundus lesions, as well as whitish chorioretinal scars, inferior-nasally. After 3 years of inflammation suppressive treatment (IST), the fundus aspect exhibited absolutely no change (A, right sex-tet). Indocyanine green angiography frames reveal numerous typical hypofluorescent dark dots (HDDs), as well as a larger hypofluorescent chorioretinal atrophic scar temporal to the fovea, before treatment (B, left 9 frames). Three years after IST, HDDs had disappeared and chorioretinal atrophy exhibited the same geographic hypofluorescent area (B, right 9 frames). This example demonstrates that HDDs do not correspond to BSRC fundus lesions, which are angiographically silent.

possibility was also demonstrated by histopathology.[23] Fuzziness of choroidal vessels indicates vasculitis of large choroidal vessels.[20] ICGA signs are present before the appearance of characteristic BSRC fundus lesions and ICGA is therefore essential for early diagnosis.[24] Most cases devoid of fundus lesions that were referred to us with vitritis and FA signs characteristic of BSRC came with a diagnosis of retinal vasculitis. Presence of both ICGA angiographic signs including HDDs and fuzziness of vessels led to HLA testing, which confirmed the diagnosis when results were positive for the HLA-A29 antigen. Both signs respond promptly to the introduction of IST; therefore ICGA is an essential modality in monitoring choroidal disease.

In several reports HDDs are thought and reported to be the angiographic expression of BSRC fundus lesions (Figure 8).[25] However, HDDs resolved in our treatment-naïve BSRC patients having fundus lesions without affecting the size or number of these fundus lesions,[18] likely because BSRC fundus lesions correspond to areas of depigmentation that no longer have any active inflammation once the stromal pigment islets have been "digested". This explains why BSRC fundus lesions are angiographically silent. Because it showed that patches of capillary leakage seen on FA, did not correspond to HDDs, ICGA also demonstrated that retinal inflammation was not related to choroidal inflammation, but occurred independent of choroidal inflammation (Figure 9).[23]

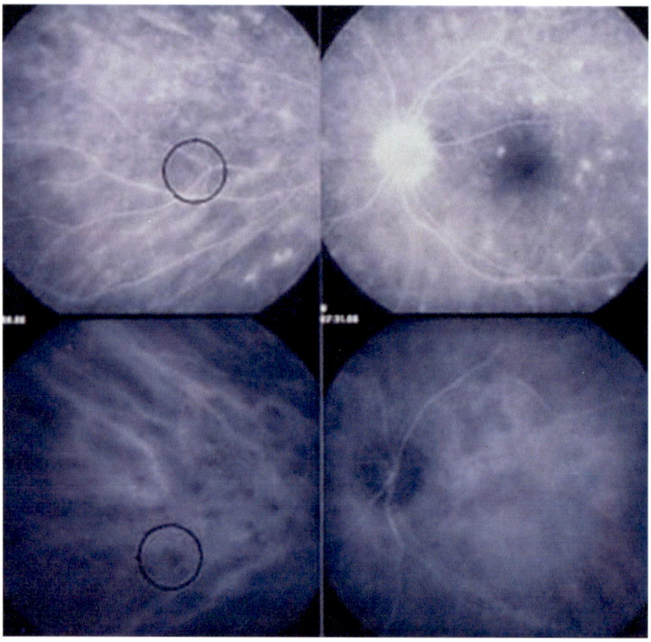

Figure 9. Retinal inflammation and choroidal inflammation are dual independent inflammatory events. The hypofluorescent dark dot encircled in the bottom left frame does not correspond to the fluorescein angiography (FA) hyperfluorescence that is visible in the same spot (top left frame.) Note, however, that the disc hyperfluorescence on FA (top right frame) also does not correspond to indocyanine green angiography (ICGA) hyperfluorescence (bottom right frame). This latter finding indicates that inflammation is not hyperacute in birdshot retinochoroidopathy, in contrast to Vogt-Koyanagi-Harada disease, for which ICGA disc hyperfluorescence is often observed.

Hypofluorescence is sometimes difficult to interpret in late disease because it can correspond to chorioretinal atrophy, in which case it will have an irregular form different from HDDs and will be hyperfluorescent on FA. Intrastromal fibrosis may be another origin of regular hypofluorescence resembling HDDs. Intrastromal fibrosis can impair ICG diffusion, and may thereby mimic disease activity. This is very rarely the case for BSRC (in contrast to VKH), because inflammation is milder and more limited for BSRC than for VKH.[26]

Visual Field Testing

In most reports on BSRC, visual acuity is the test used to monitor function. This does not seem to be appropriate because visual acuity can be preserved for a prolonged period, while dimness of vision and subjective visual field disturbance can be very pronouced. We showed in 1999 that this subjective visual disturbance was associated with visual field changes and that visual field monitoring allowed the assessment of treatment efficacy.[27] In a recent report we showed that all patients diagnosed with BSRC presented visual field disturbance, without exception.[18] One patient presented with bilateral tubular visual fields with a bilateral vision of 1.0 (20/20). This patient complained of severe peripheral field impairment that recovered substantially after introduction of IST (Figure 10). The importance of visual field testing has been increasingly recognized in the last few years.[28] In one report the rate of visual field disturbance amounted to 100%, as in our series.[29] The presence of visual field changes in nearly 100% of patients might qualify this functional test not only for monitoring purposes but also as a diagnostic criterion.

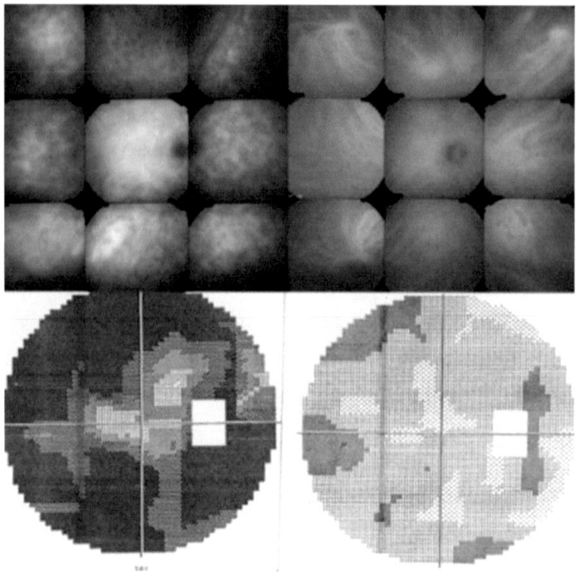

Figure 10. Severe visual field changes without loss of visual acuity. This patient was seen 9 months after the onset of symptoms and complained of dimness of vision and subjective visual field impairment. Octopus® perimetry revealed tubular visual fields bilaterally (bottom left, right eye shown), severe retinitis on fluorescein angiography (not shown), as well as numerous hypofluorescent dark dots and fuzziness of choroidal vessels (top left set of 9 frames) . After inflammation suppressive treatment (IST), the indocyanine green angiography choroidal aspect was restored to a quasi-normal condition (top right set of 9 frames) and the patient's visual field recovered substantially (bottom right, right eye shown).

Electrophysiology

If available, electrophysiology is another investigational procedure that can be useful to localize disease impact and to monitor disease progression. In an early study on electroretinogram (ERG) in BSC, Priem et al. suggested that dysfunction resides in the inner retina, which corroborates FA and OCT findings that show diffuse retinal edema from diffusely leaking retinal capillaries (of which the functional counterpart is visual field changes).[30] ERG data by Holder et al. also indicate that function of the inner retina is impaired.[31] These authors also showed that ERG improves after the initiation of treatment; it could therefore be considered a reliable method for monitoring treatment efficacy.

HLA Testing

Association of BSRC with the HLA-A29 tissue histocompatibility antigen was first reported in 1982, 2 years after the entity was originally described.[6] The association rate was estimated to be approximately 95% in different subsequent reports.[32,33] LeHoang et al. found that BSRC was associated with the HLA-A29-2 subtype,[34] which was later put in doubt.[35] It becomes increasingly likely that the association is closer to 100%, as false negatives are not so rare when the antibody testing method is used. The rate of false negative results can be reduced when PCR-based testing is used.[36] Truly HLA-A29-negative birdshot patients are a rarity if they exist at all and limiting the diagnosis to PCR-positive HLA-A29 patients would exclude a tiny proportion of patients, if any patients at all. Therefore, presence of HLA-A29 antigen should be an essential criterion for the diagnosis of BSRC allowing inclusion in clinical trials.

DIAGNOSTIC CRITERIA

In 2006 a group of experts published research criteria for the diagnosis of BSRC.[4] However, these criteria fail to truly characterize BSRC, especially early-stage disease. The major shortcomings are the omission of ICGA signs, which are present in nearly 100% of cases; lack of any reference to the visual field changes that are present in almost 100% of cases; the characterization of HLA-A29 antigen as merely a supporting factor even though it is present in almost 100% of cases; and finally the lack of acknowledgment that KPs cannot be an exclusion criterion as they are present in close to 20% of treatment-naïve patients. There is an urgent need for new and proper criteria for the correct appraisal and management of BSRC. In our studies we used following criteria: presence of vitritis and retinal vasculitis in one or both eyes, visual field anomalies in one or both eyes, stromal choroiditis as evidenced by ICGA in both eyes, presence of HLA-A29 antigen positivity and absence of extra-ocular inflammation sites. An additional (but not obligatory) criterion was the presence of rice-shaped, depigmented "birdshot lesions" (BSRC fundus lesions).

TREATMENT AND DISEASE PROGRESSION

Treatment Guidelines

For many years after BSRC was described, the opinion prevailed that BSRC did not necessarily require aggressive IST administration.[37-39] The reason for such a position was twofold: (1) early reports had placed the efficacy of IST in doubt and (2) the functional criterion used to follow disease evolution was visual acuity, which we now know to be inappropriate because central vision remains excellent in a substantial proportion of patients, even after years of disease progression.[40]

There is increasing evidence that aggressive and sustained treatment is probably needed in the majority of patients;[41,42] no more than 10% to 15% of patients present a relatively mild course.[8] Once the diagnosis is established, our criterion to treat is the occurrence of visual field defects. If involvement is unilateral, then the introduction of systemic immunosuppressive treatment can sometimes be deferred for a period of time by using sub-Tenon's injections of triamcinolone acetonide (40 mg per injection) every 4–6 months if the other eye is not functionally affected. Once systemic treatment is decided, our regimen combines systemic or sub-Tenon's steroids with immunosuppressants, mostly mycophenolic acid (Myfortic®). Steroids are subsequently tapered to 0 or to <7.5 mg per day. In case of insufficient recovery of visual fields and/or persistence of retinal inflammatory signs (mainly monitored by FA), a second immunosuppressant or biologic agent is added (e.g., anti-TNF-α antibodies). We demonstrated that substantial improvement of visual field parameters and maintenance of central vision can be obtained, as well as resolution of ICGA and improvement of FA signs.[18] Early treatment is usually the rule. However, at present treatment is too often delayed because of a delayed diagnosis or because patients decline treatment. We showed that insufficient or delayed treatment results in retinal atrophy, as evidenced by OCT.[19]

Early Treatment Changes the Clinical Phenotype of BSRC

We recently showed that, among patients that were treated before the development of BSRC fundus lesions, the appearance of such lesions could be prevented in 5 of 6 patients treated within a mean of 6.5 months of symptoms and observed during a mean period of 10 years of treatment.[8] In this regard BSRC behaved like VKH, another stromal choroiditis in which it has also been shown that early, vigorous and prolonged treatment can prevent the development of sunset glow fundus (Figure 11).[43] Indeed, such prevention of BSRC fundus lesions requires early diagnosis, which is not possible with the present diagnostic criteria.

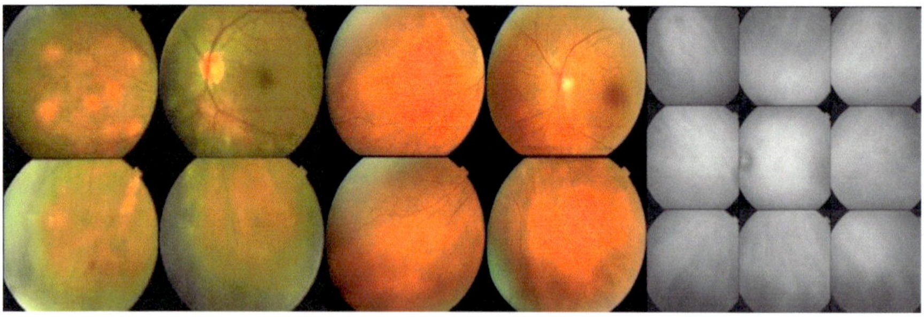

Figure 11. Early treatment can change the phenotype of birdshot retinochoroidopathy (BSRC). This woman was 54 years old at presentation; her history featured a 42-month diagnostic delay and a 48-month treatment delay (left eye). Fundus images taken at presentation (left quartet of images) reveal typical BSRC fundus lesions that regressed after 10 years of inflammation suppressive treatment (IST) to leave faint discoloration (center quartet) that do not meet the research criteria for the diagnosis of BSRC. After 10 years of IST, indocyanine green angiography (right set of 9 frames) reveals absence of hypofluorescent dark dots.

Conclusions

Birdshot retinochoroidopathy is a granulomatous ocular inflammatory disease that seems to be limited to the eye. It appears to lack any known extraocular site of inflammation and demonstrates nearly 100% association with the leukocyte histocompatibility antigen HLA-A29. Dual parallel non-related inflammation of the retina and the choroid is particular to BSRC. Retinal involvement is responsible for substantial clinical morbidity if the disease is left untreated. Treatment (IST) must be started early and should be vigorous and prolonged.

Choroidal involvement responds rather well and rapidly to IST; the development of depigmented BSRC fundus lesions can even be prevented if treatment is started early. The impact of therapy on retinal disease is more limited but can likely avoid retinal atrophy if treatment is applied early. However, ICGA is crucial to achieve early diagnosis before the appearance of what has thus far been considered the hallmark of BSRC: rice-shaped choroidal depigmented fundus lesions.

Take-home messages

- Birdshot retinochoroidopathy (BSRC) is an intraocular inflammatory disease that features two independent inflammatory events: severe retinitis and stromal choroiditis.

- Retinal disease is subdivided into two stages: early exudative and late atrophic, and is at the origin of the preponderant part of disease morbidity.
- The early exudative stage of the retina is going over to a late atrophic stage if insufficiently treated and thus causes major functional impairment.
- The trigger of stromal choroiditis is situated in the stromal melanocyte islets, although the antigen remains unknown.
- Birdshot retinochoroidopathy is a granulomatous uveitis that can present with KPs.
- Fluorescein angiography (FA) provides the best analysis of retinal involvement, including retinal exudation from small to large retinal vessels, which can cause diffuse retinal edema in the exudative phase, vascular sheathing and disc hyperfluorescence.
- The fovea is relatively spared from the massive retinal edema, which explains the good visual acuity retained by a relatively large proportion of patients during a relatively long period.
- Indocyanine green angiography (ICGA), which is crucial to the analysis of choroidal disease, shows numerous hypofluorescent dark dots (HDDs) and fuzziness of large choroidal vessels. The HDDs are produced by stromal inflammatory foci and choroidal vessel fuzziness indicates choroidal vasculitis.
- ICGA is able to reveal active stromal choroiditis, which is always occult.
- ICGA is necessary to diagnose early disease before the appearance of BSRC fundus lesions.

- Choroidal disease only becomes apparent later when hypo/depigmented rice-shaped fundus lesions can be observed.
- Occult HDDs do not correspond to BSRC fundus lesions that have no translation on ICGA.
- Visual field testing should be used as the main functional parameter.
- HLA-A29 antigen is positive in almost 100% of patients and represents the strongest diagnostic criterion in the presence of a compatible clinical picture.
- In >85% of BSRC patients, aggressive and sustained inflammation suppressive treatment (IST) is necessary. This treatment can comprise one or two immunosuppressants and/or biologicals administered early in disease so long as functional (visual field) impairment is present.
- If administered early (i.e., before BSRC depigmented fundus lesions appear), IST can modify the disease phenotype by preventing the appearance of such lesions.

References

1. Gasch, AT, Smith JA, Whitcup SM. Birdshot retinochoroidopathy. Br J Ophthalmol, 1999. 83:241-9.
2. Ryan, SJ and AE Maumenee, *Birdshot retinochoroidopathy*. Am J Ophthalmol, 1980. 89:31-45.
3. Gass JDM. Vitiliginous chorioretinitis. Arch Ophthalmol1981; 99:1778-87.
4. Levinson RD, Brezin A, Rothova A, et al.. Research criteria for the diagnosis of birdshot chorioretinopathy: results of an international consensus conference. Am J Ophthalmol 2006; 141: 185-7.
5. Guex-Crosier Y, Herbort CP. Prolonged retinal arterio-venous circulation time by fluorescein but not by indocyanine green angiography in birdshot chorioretinopathy. Ocul Immunol Inflamm, 1997. 5:203-6.
6. Nussenblatt RB, Mittal KK, Ryan S, et al.Birdshot retinochoroidopathy associated with HLA-A29 antigen and immune responsiveness to retinal S-antigen. Am J Ophthalmol 1982; 94:147-58.
7. Gaudio PA, Kaye DB, Crawford JB. Histopathology of birdshot retinochoroidopathy. Br J Ophthalmol 2002; 86:1439-41.
8. Papadia M, Knecht PB, Herbort CP. Early and sustained treatment modifies the phenotype of birdshot retinochoroidopathy. Acta Ophthalmologica 2013; 91, s252: DOI 10 1111/j 1755-3768.2013.x.
9. Knecht PB, Papadia M, Herbort CP. Granulomatous keratic precipitates in birdshot retinochoroidopathy. Int Ophthalmol 2013; 33:133-7.

10. Guex-Crosier Y, Pittet N, Herbort CP. Sensitivity of laser flare photometryto monitor inflammation in uveitis of the posterior segment. Ophthalmology 1995; 102:613-621.
11. Monnet D, Brézin A, Holland GN, et al.. Longitudinal cohort study of patients with birdshot chorioretinopathy. I. Baseline clinical charcteristics. Am J Ophthalmol 2006; 141:135-142.
12. Herbort CP, LeHoang P, Guex-Crosier Y. Schematic interpretation of indocyanine green angiography in posterior uveitis using a standard angiographic protocol. Ophthalmology 1998; 105:432-40.
13. Herbort CP. Posterior uveitis: new insights provided by indocanine green angiography. Eye 1998; 12:757-9.
14. Bouchenaki N, Herbort CP. Stromal choroiditis. In: Pleyer U, Mondino B eds. Essentials in Ophthalmology: Uveitis and Immunological Disorders. Berlin, Heidelberg,New York : Springer, 2004; pp 234-253.
15. Sugita S, Takase H, Taguchi C, et al. Ocular infiltrating CD4+ T cells from patients with Vogt-Koyanagi-Harada disease recognize human melanocyte antigens. Invest Ophthalmol Vis Sci 2006; 47:2547-54.
16. Herbort CP, Mantovani A, Bouchenaki N. Indocyanine green angiography in Vogt-Koyanagi-Harada disease: angiographic signs and utility in patient follow-up. Int Ophthalmol 2007; 27:173-82.
17. Herbort CP, Probst K, Cimino L, Tran VT. Differential inflammatory involvement in retina and choroid in birdshot chorioretinopathy. Klin Monbl Augenheilkd, 2004; 221: 351-6.
18. Papadia M, Herbort CP. Reappraisal of birdshot retinochoroidopathy (BSRC): a global approach. Graefe's Arch Clin Exp Ophthalmol 2013; 251:861-9.

19. Papadia M, Jeannin B, Herbort CP. OCT findings in birdshot chorioretinitis: a glimpse into retinal disease evolution. Ophthalmic Surg Lasers Imaging 2012; 43-suppl S25-31.
20. Herbort CP, Mantovani A, Papadia M. Use of indocyanine green angiography in uveitis. Int Ophthalmol Clin 2012; 52:13-31.
21. Herbort CP, Neri P, Abu El Asrar AA, et al. Is ICGA still relevant in inflammatory eye disorders? Why this question has to be dealt with separately from other eye conditions. Retina 2012; 32:1701-3.
22. Herbort CP, Papadia M, Mantovani A. Classification of choroiditis based on inflammatory lesion process rather than fundus appearance: enhanced comprehensionthrough the ICGA concepts of the iceberg and jellyfish effects. Lin Monbl Augenheilk 2012; 229:306-13.
23. Fardeau C, Herbort CP, Kullmann N, et al. Indocyanine green angiography in birdshot chorioretinopathy. Ophthalmology, 1999. 106:1928-34.
24. Papadia M, Herbort CP. Indocyanine green angiography (ICGA) is essential for the early diagnosis of birdshot chorioretinopathy. Klin Monbl Augenheilkd 2012; 229:348-52.
25. Leder HA, Galor A, Thorne JE, Jabs D. Disappearance of classic birdshot spots after immunosuppression with tacrolimus and mycophenolate mofetyl. Br J Ophthalmol 2008; 92:291.
26. Knecht PB, Mantovani A, Herbort CP. Indocyanine green angiography-guided management of Vogt-Koyanagi-Harada disease. Int Ophthalmol 2013; Jan 1 (Epub ahead of print)

27. de Courten C, Herbort CP. Potential role of computerized visual field testing for the appraisal and follow-up of birdshot chorioretinopathy. Arch Ophthalmol 1998; 116:1389-91.
28. Thorne JE, Jabs DA, Kedhar SR, et al.. Loss of visual field among patients with birdshot chorioretinopathy. Am J Ophthalmol 2008; 145:23-28.
29. Gordon LK, Monnet D, Holland GN, et al.. Longitudinal cohort study of patients with birdshot chorioretinopathy. IV. Visual field. Am J Ophthalmol 2007; 144:829-37.
30. Priem HA, De Rouck A, De Laey JJ, Bird AC. Electrophysiologic studies in birdshot chorioretinopathy. Am J Ophthalmol 1988; 106:430-6.
31. Holder GE, Robson AG, Pavésio C, Graham EM. Electrophysiological characterization and monitoring in the management of birdshot chorioretinopathy. Br J Ophthalmol 2005; 88:709-18.
32. Baarsma GS, Priem HA, Kijlstra A. Association of birdshot retinochoroidopathy and HLA-A29 antigen. Curr Eye Res. 1990; 9-Suppl.:63-8.
33. Brezin AP, Monnet D, Cohen JH, Levinson RD. HLA-A29 and birdshot chorioretinopathy. Ocul Immunol Inflamm 2011; 19:397-400.
34. LeHoang P, Osdemir N, Benhamou A, et al. HLA-A29.2 subtype associated with birdshot retinochoroidopathy. Am J Ophthalmol 1992; 113:33-5.
35. Levinson RD, Rajalingam R, Park MS, et al. Human leukocyte antigen A29 subtypes associated with birdshot retinochoroidopathy. Am J Ophthalmol 2004; 138:631-4.
36. Wender JD, Fu AD, Jumper JM, et al. False-negative antibody-based HLA-A29 typing in two patients with birdshot chorioretinopathy. Br J Ophthalmol 2008; 92:1153-4.

37. Priem HA, Oosterhuis JA. Birdshot chorioretinopathy: clinical characteristics and evolution. Br J Ophthalmol 1988; 72 : 646-59.
38 The American Academy of Ophthalmology Basic and Clinical Science Course, The Foundation of the American Academy of Ophthalmology, San Francisco (Pub.), Volume 9, Intraocular Inflammation and uveitis, 2000-2001 Edition, pp 170-1.
39. Nussenblatt RB, Wuitcup SM, Palestine AG. Birdshot retinochoroidopathy. In Uveitis, Fundamentals and Clinical Practice, second edition. St.-Louis , Mosby 1996; pp 325-333.
40. Rothova A, Berendschot TTJM, Probst K, et al.. Birdshot Chorioretinopathy, long-term manifestations and visual prognosis. Ophthalmology 2004; 111:954-9.
41. Kiss S, Ahmed M, Leiko E, Foster CS. Long-term follow-up of patients with birdshot retinochoroidopathy treated with corticosteroid-sparing systemic immunomodulatory therapy. Ophthalmology 2005; 112:1066-71.
42. Cervantes-Castaneda RA, Gonzalez-Gonzalez LA, Cordero-Coma M, et al. Combined therapy of cyclosporine A and mycophenolate mofetil for the treatment of birdshot retinochoroidopathy : a 12-month follow-up. Br J Ophthalmol 2013; 97:637-43.
43. Bouchenaki N, Herbort CP. Indocyanine green angiography guided management of Vogt-Koyanagi-Harada disease. J Ophthalmic Vis Res. 6:241-8.

Chapter 9

Determinants of Remission and Cure

Phuc LeHoang

The chronic intraocular inflammation seen in birdshot retinochoroidopathy is responsible for progressive and severe retinal dysfunction in the majority of the patients despite iterative therapeutic attempts. To improve the visual outcome, it is essential to analyze the possible determinants of remissions and cure that can guide the monitoring and the treatment, particularly since there is no known standardized therapeutic regimen for controlling the disease. Thus one should try to set (1) the criteria by which one can warrant a remission or a cure, and to seek for (2) the factors associated with a bad prognosis, and (3) the factors linked with a better visual outcome. Although the individualization of the majority of those factors is biased and may vary substantially from one study to the other, it appears that an aggressive treatment is essential for eradicating any subclinical low-grade inflammation responsible of the severe visual prognosis of birdshot.

Introduction

Because birdshot retinochoroidopathy (BSRC) is a sight-threatening condition with a relentless, long duration progressive course and unpredictable exacerbations,[1,2,3,4,5,6] it appears essential to set determinants of remission and cure. Those determinants will help to guide physician action for each individual patient, whatever the stage of the disease may be. As the disease evolves over a long period of time (20-30 years), the establishment of the level of inflammatory activity along with a very close monitoring can help the ophthalmologist in adjusting the therapeutic regimen and therefore in inflecting the natural course of the inevitable progressive visual loss if the patients are left untreated or insufficiently treated.

There is no standardized treatment for this rare disease.[7, 8] The determinants of remissions and cure can minimize groping for the adequate choice of drugs provided that each proposed therapeutic regimen is assessed shortly after its initiation. Determinants include two components: (1) the criteria by which one can state that the patient is in remission or is cured and (2) the criteria enabling to predict the course of the disease progressing towards either remission or worsening.

DEFINITIONS

***Remission**:* The state of absence of disease activity in patients with a chronic illness, with the possibility of return of disease activity. Remission is a period of time when the disease is responding to treatment or is under control.

In a complete remission, all the signs and symptoms of the disease disappear. It is also possible for a patient to have a partial remission in which the inflammation subsides but does not completely disappear.

Remissions can last anywhere from several weeks to many years. According to the SUN criteria,[9] a remission is defined as an inactive disease for ≥ 3 months after discontinuing all treatments for eye disease. However, this definition seems inadequate for the BSRC patients who can suffer from unpredictable exacerbations with a "wax and wane" type of course that can last several decades. A more pragmatic approach would be an absence of disease activity for at least 1 to 2 years for describing a remission in BSRC.

Some complete remissions may last for years and may be considered as cures.

If the disease returns, another remission often can occur with further treatment. An inflammation that has recurred may respond to a different type of therapy, including a different drug combination.

***Cure**:* A cure is the end of a medical condition. All the signs and symptoms of the disease must disappear off medication. It is exceptionally spontaneous (as for a common cold). It occurs more often after an adequate treatment. The required period of time needed to state that a patient is cured is variable according to the type of disease: it can vary from two to ten years.

Because the occurrence and the duration of the cured state is unpredictable, one often refers to a "cure rate". A 5-year cure rate of 70% corresponds to a 5-year remission in 70% of the cases.

Two questions worry the uveitis specialist: Firstly, how can we define remission and cure in BSRC; what criteria may we use? Secondly, what factors can determine or predict the occurrence of a remission or a cure during the course of the disease?

How We Can Define Remission and Cure in BSRC

1. Complete remission on medication: all the following criteria must be under control with an adequate therapeutic regimen.

- Clinical criteria:
    - Visual acuity: stabilized or improved visual acuity. Subjective symptoms and clinical signs - and especially visual acuity - are poor indicators of generalized retinal function in BSRC.

- No anterior segment inflammation
  - Vitreous cells: no or trace cells
  - No active fluffy retinal vasculitis
  - No macular edema
  - No optic disc edema
- Ancillary tests
  - Quiet FA (no vasculitis leakage, no choriocapillaris hyperfluorescence, no optic disk leakage)
  - Quiet ICG-A *(no dark spots, no choroidal vessel dilation, no late hyperfluorescence of the post pole)*
  - OCT: No active macular edema, no active cystoid macular edema, stabilization or improvement of the IS/OS layer alterations.
  - Stabilized or improved visual fields (Humphrey, Goldmann)
  - ERG: Stabilization of electrophysiological abnormalities, particularly stabilized or improved ERG 30Hz implicit times.
- Visual field and electrophysiological assessments are quantifiable.

Repeated visual field and electrophysiological assessments provide objective and reliable measures for monitoring disease activity and are essential to testify a complete remission, there is evidence that a chronic progressive retinal dysfunction, measured by Goldmann or Humphrey visual field testing or by electroretinography, may occur even in the absence of evident vitritis and CME and in the presence of a normal central visual acuity.[4,6,10,11]

Electrophysiological assessment can demonstrate improvement following treatment. It can therefore evaluate therapeutic efficacy and allows an adjustment of therapy leading to improved long term prognosis.[12,13,14,15]

2. Possible definitions of partial remission for BSRC

Following is a typical picture of an insufficiently treated patient:

- Stabilized visual acuity
- Persistent creeping insidious activity:
    - Progressing ERG alterations
    - Slow visual field deterioration
    - Mild vitritis, floaters
    - FA: persistence of hyperfluorescence of the choriocapillaris despite the absence of vascular leakage or cystoid macular edema
    - ICG-A: few persistent scarce dark hypofluorescent dots
    - Choroidal neovascularization
    - Mild macular edema on OCT

Because the (1) choroidal inflammation, the (2) inner and (3) outer retinal dysfunction may occur independently,[3] one of those three components may still be active whereas the two others are apparently stabilized or improved. In the presence of an apparent clinical inactivity of the disease (stabilized or improved visual acuity, visual field, vitritis, symptoms), if one or two of the three components remain active, the remission may be considered as partial.

This is what happens in most cases, related to the insufficient treatment administered to the patients and explaining the severe visual dysfunction at later stages of the disease. Relying only on inadequate criteria (symptoms, visual acuity, visual fields, vitritis, FA and ICG-A features, gross OCT analysis without high resolution examination) can lead to an insufficient and unsatisfying treatment.

Patients may present with (1) either a "quiet" FA (no leakage from the retinal vessels or capillaries, the choriocapillaris, the optic disc, no macular edema) with an active choroidal disease with persistent hypofluorescent spots on the ICG-A, or, even more frequently, (2) the reverse. As the choroidal disease is more readily responsive to the treatment than the creeping retinal disease, one must not overlook a persistent inflammatory activity by considering only one of the monitoring criteria.

As stated above, one must check all the monitoring criteria, one by one, before considering a remission for the patient and therefore before tapering the treatment dosage.

3. Durable remission off medication:

One can artificially differentiate clinical remission on medication (6 continuous months of inactive disease on medication) from clinical durable remission off medication (12 months of inactive disease off all medications).

BSRC is wrongly considered as a chronically progressive disease resistant to treatment. An aggressive use of corticosteroids can control the inflammatory exacerbations and must be combined with early immunomodulatory therapy (IMT) that will further help to control the inflammation and allow tapering of corticosteroids dosage.[16]

Long-term preservation of visual function is attainable with systemic corticosteroid-sparing IMT for patients suffering from BSRC.[17] The control of inflammation can be achieved with a minimal maintenance treatment.

In some patients treated with immunomodulatory therapy (IMT), a durable remission is achievable after discontinuation of therapy. In case of durable remission, the absence of inflammation without any systemic IMT should last for at least 1 year.

In a retrospective study, 50 (among them, four were BSRC patients) out of 399 patients suffering from various ocular inflammatory diseases treated with systemic IMT for a period of two to five years showed a durable remission. between two and five years in 20% of the cases and 18% were in remission for more than five years after treatment discontinuation. Those durable remissions may be considered as a five-year cure rate.[18]

Among 40 BSRC patients treated with a combination of cyclosporine A and mycophenolate mofetil, 27% had a durable remission off IMT and 29% had a clinical remission on long-term IMT.[3] Durable remission off treatment is therefore an attainable and realistic goal and can be considered as a cure of the disease.

Early and aggressive treatment with systemic IMT may offer the best hope of maintaining retinal function in what is often thought of as a chronically progressive disease resistant to treatment.

4. Cure

Cure would imply that the disease has been inactive without treatment for a long period of time which should be determined: a five- to ten-year period seems preferable but a two-year period can be considered reasonable.

Cure is rare but may still be attainable. Cure must not be confused with a burned out end stage disease with no more inflammatory activity and a severe visual impairment compromising an acceptable life.

- Cure:
  - No active inflammation off medication for at least 2 years.
  - Good remaining visual function
  - No severe sequelae
- Burned-out:
  - No active inflammation
  - Severe visual impairment
    - *Retinal atrophy, vessel narrowing, pigmentary loss*
    - *Optic atrophy*

What Factors Can Determine the Occurrence of Remission or Cure During the Course of the Disease?[6,12,16,18,19]

- Early Rx: *Early introduction of IMT*
- Normal or subnormal EOG *(Arden's ratio, mean maximal amplitude value of electric potential)*
- Partial recovery of 30 Hz flicker implicit time on Rx
- Stabilization or improvement of Visual Fields (Humphrey and particularly Goldmann testings)
- Restoration of Retinal Architecture (SD-OCT) following Systemic Immunosuppression
- Clinical features were not reliable indicators of functional deterioration or recovery.

Determinants for a poor prognosis:

- Clinical features:
    - Longer time interval between the initial symptoms and the diagnosis
    - A longer duration of the disease is associated with poorer visual outcomes.
    - Retinal vasculitis
    - CME
- Ancillary test features
    - Severe visual fields alterations

    - OCT: loss, alterations, disruption of the IS/OS junction, disorganization of the inner retinal layers, photoreceptors and RPE atrophy, macular/foveal atrophy, hyper-refflective material in the outer nuclear layer, decreased choroidal thickness,
    - FAF: placoid macular hypofluorescence indicative of RPE atrophy
    - Mf ERG: reduced overall and foveal response density
- Inadequate therapeutic regimen associated with a poor outcome.
    - Long term treatment with systemic corticosteroids alone. In the vast majority of the patients, high doses of steroids are necessary to control the intraocular inflammation and are not tolerable leading to a decrease of steroids dosage to an acceptable level which is insufficient to control the progressive retinal dysfunction. Long term follow-up of patients primarily treated with steroids showed poor visual outcomes.
    - No early initiation of IMT. At this time, the only way to permit an adequate control of the intraocular inflammation is to start the IMT as early as necessary. A cautious strategy would be to initiate the IMT as soon as the level of the corticosteroids tapering become ineffective to prevent the development of the disease. One can start the IMT when the level of steroid dependence is reached.

However, most of the uveitis specialists acquainted with the management of BSRC tend to initiate the IMT earlier in the course, either from the very beginning or as soon as the inflammation is controlled by the corticosteroids whatever the steroid dosage is, thus enabling a sooner and easier steroids tapering in order to avoid long term corticosteroids adverse effects. By acting on more specific components of the immune and inflammatory responses than the steroids monotherapy, the IMT can better control the various mechanisms of the immune mediated disease and may achieve durable remission.

Small preliminary study at Pitie-Salpetriere Hospital (56 BSRC patients: We attempt to bring out clinical factors that can determine the outcome of the disease. This small retrospective study includes 56 BSRC patients with a follow-up of at least 2 years. Mean followup was 12.5 ± 4.9 years from the onset of symptoms.

We observed the following distribution of outcomes:

- *Partial remission = 20*
- *Complete remission on medication = 19*
- *Worsening = 15*
- *« Cured » off medication = 2*

Factors associated with a deterioration of visual function:

- Slightly younger patients
- History of cardiovascular or cerebrovascular accident
- History of autoimmune conditions
- Initial visual acuity < 20/40
- Initial Retinal vasculitis
- late CME during the course
- Initial 10-2 HVF MD < -10
- Longer time interval between the occurrence of the initial symptoms and the introduction of IMT

Factors associated with a higher chance to achieve clinical remission and with a better prognosis

- Initial Vitritis ≥ 2 +
- CME at initial assessment
- Choroidal spots on initial ICG angiographic assessment
- Fluorescein Leakage at initial angiographic assessment
- EOG mean amplitude maximal value at initial assessment

The paradoxical finding that initial vitritis, fluorescein leakage and CME were associated with a better outcome may be explained by the fact that a more aggressive initial treatement was administered in the presence of obvious significant inflammatory activity. It appears that an aggressive treatment is essential for eradicating any subclinical low-grade inflammation responsible of the severe visual prognosis of BSRC.

Thus, the individualization of the majority of those factors is biased and may vary substantially from one retrospective study to the other. They depend upon the stage of the disease at the initial visit, the previous and ongoing treatment, the consistency of the monitoring, the stubbornness of finding alternative therapies.

Proposed Strategy to achieve Remission and Cure

1. Therapeutic strategy[3,6,17]

- Progressive diffuse retinal dysfunction is an important cause of visual impairment.
- The goal is to achieve quiescence through aggressive use of corticosteroids to extinguish the fire and then move along to achieve steroid-free remission through immunosuppressant agents.
- Early introduction of chronic prolonged immunosuppressive drug
    - ✓ *reduces the risk of developing visual impairment and structural ocular complications, independent of previous oral corticosteroid therapy.*

- ✓ *allows tapering of prednisone to an acceptable level*
- ✓ *and may improve long-term outcomes in BSRC*

- Patients with active inflammation are maintained on systemic IMT until the disease has remained quiescent for 2 years, after which medications are slowly tapered.

Corticosteroid-sparing Systemic IMT [20,21,22]

- *Cyclosporine, MMF, AZA, MTX*
- *Biologics : IvIg, IFN, Anti-TNF (Infliximab, Adalimumab), Daclizumab (anti-IL-2R alpha), Tocilizumab (anti-soluble and membrane bound IL-6 Rrs)*
- *Combined therapy +++ (AZA+CSA; CSA+MMF)*

Corticosteroids monotherapy confers a misleading security

- Corticosteroids may be used to control recent active inflammation but are insufficient to prevent the progressive retinal alterations occurring during the chronic course of the disease at acceptable dosage.
- Natural history of BSRC or the outcomes with corticosteroid therapy alone, showed a persistent worsening of vision with time despite an apparent clinical remission. [4,5,7,23,24,25]

2. Adequate Monitoring Strategy:

One should perform a very close monitoring with repeated short time interval visits.

Short term monitoring

Clinical examination and ancillary tests : FA, ICG-A, OCT participate to the short term evaluation of the intraocular inflammation.

However, one should not rely on the measurement of visual acuity for the therapeutic management, as visual acuity is an inadequate tool for determining when to treat.[12,26] When the decision to treat was based on loss of Snellen visual acuity or vascular leakage on fluorescein angiograms, treatment appeared to be ineffective in arresting worsening of vision. The visual symptoms are often disproportionate to clinical findings and measured visual acuity (VA). Patients are often complaining of vision loss despite no change in measured VA (nyctalopia, dyschromatopsia, photopsia), because there is a tendency for subclinical insidious progression with preservation of the visual acuity in many patients.

Long term monitoring

The long term monitoring should rely on objective measures, such as ERGs and visual field testing, that can orientate management decisions with early initiatin or modification of treatment. Subjective symptoms and clinical signs are poor indicators of generalized retinal function in BSRC [12,13].

Monitor ERGs: Abnormalities are usually present in the electroretinograms (ERGs) of these patients, including decreased scotopic and photopic amplitudes and delay in the 30-hertz (Hz) flicker implicit time of the electrical responses, indicative of early stage retinal dysfunction.

Electrophysiological examination provides a method of monitoring the efficacy of treatment, and may facilitate therapeutic decisions and may lead to improved long term prognosis.

No patient had sufficient control of BSRC with corticosteroid therapy without IMT. Patients treated with steroids alone show progressive ERG decline.

The presence of a normal 30 Hz response in BCR following treatment has been reported as a good prognostic sign, allowing tapering of IMT without rebound inflammation. Normalized retinal function can be achieved in BCR following.

Serial Visual Field tests are another potentially useful ancillary test for following up BSRC. Automated and Goldmann visual field testing provide objective measures of disease activity such as ERG testing. The use of IMT may reverse some of the visual field alterations.[4,7,10,27]

SD-OCT and High resolution Depth Enhanced OCT [19,26,28,29]

OCT technology allows a very detailed analysis of retinal structures. It can show IS/OS layer alterations that may be reversible on efficient treatment.

Conclusion

The remission on or off medication is attainable providing:

1. A close monitoring with short interval visits

The first line or short term monitoring correspond to the usual uveitis monitoring procedure (symptoms, clinical examination, fluorescein and ICG angiograms, OCT ...). Visual acuity measurement is not a reliable indicator of the disease activity and may remain normal despite a progressive retinal dysfunction.

The second line or long term monitoring comprises ERG (30Hz flicker ERG implicit times) and visual fields (automated or Goldmann) testing enabling to refine the therapeutic strategy.

2. An aggressive treatment that should be continuously evaluated and adjusted for suppressing any residual inflammation no matter how low it is. There is a need for an early diagnosis and an early treatment. One should introduce early systemic IMT and prohibit intermittent treatment and periocular corticosteroids as a sole therapy.

References

1. Opremcak EM. (1994) Birdshot retinochoroidopathy. In: Albert DM, Jakobiec FA, eds. Principles and Practice of Ophthalmology: Clinical Practice. Vol. 1. (475–80) Philadelphia: WB Saunders.
2. LeHoang P, Ryan SJ. (1996) Birdshot Retinochoroidopathy. In: Pepose JS, Holland GN, Wilhelmus KR, eds. Ocular Infection and Immunity. (570-578) St Louis: Mosby.
3. Vitale AT (2013). Birdshot Retinochoroidopathy. In CS Foster & AT Vitale eds, Diagnosis and Treatment of Uveitis (pp. 982-1004). New Delhi, India, Jaypee Brothers Medical Publishers.
4. Oh KT, Christmas NJ, Folk JC. Birdshot retinochoroidopathy: long term follow-up of a chronically progressive disease. Am J Ophthalmol 2002;133:622–9.
5. Rothova A, Berendschot TT, Probst K, et al. Birdshot retinochoroidopathy: long-term manifestations and visual prognosis. Ophthalmology 2004;111:954 –9.
6. Thorne JE, Jabs DA, Peters GB, Hair D, Dunn JP, Kempen JH. Birdshot retinochoroidopathy: ocular complications and visual impairment. *Am J Ophthalmol.* 2005;140(1):45-51.
7. Gasch AT, Smith JA, Whitcup SM. Birdshot retinochoroidopathy. Br J Ophthalmol 1999;83:241–9.
8. Quillen DA, Davis JB, Gottlieb JL, et al. The white dot syndromes. Am J Ophthalmol 2004;137:538 –50.

9. Jabs DA, Nussenblatt RB, Rosenbaum JT; Standardization of Uveitis Nomenclature (SUN) Working Group. Standardization of uveitis nomenclature for reporting clinical data. Results of the First International Workshop. Am J Ophthalmol. 2005: 140(3):509-16.
10. Thorne JE, Jabs DA, Kedhar SR et al. Loss of Visual Field Among Patients with Birdshot Retinochoroidopathy. Am J Ophthalmol 2008;145:23–28.
11. Gordon LK, Monnet D, Holland GN et al. Longitudinal Cohort Study of Patients with Birdshot Retinochoroidopathy. IV. Visual Field Results at Baseline. Am J Ophthalmol 2007;144:829–837.
12. Holder GE, Robson AG, Pavesio C, Graham EM. Electrophysiological characterisation and monitoring in the management of birdshot retinochoroidopathy. Br J Ophthalmol 2005;89:709–718.
13. Sobrin L, Lam BL, Liu M, Feuer WJ, Davis JL. Electroretinographic monitoring in birdshot retinochoroidopathy. Am J Ophthalmol 2005;140:52–64.
14. Zacks DN, Samson CM, Loewenstein J, Foster CS. Electroretinograms as an indicator of disease activity in birdshot retinochoroidopathy. Graefe's Arch Clin Exp Ophthalmol 2002;240:601– 607.
15. Birch DG, Williams PD, Callanan D et al. Macular atrophy in birdshot retinochoroidopathy: an optical coherence tomography and multifocal electroretinography analysis. Retina. 2010;30(6):930-937.
16. Siddique SS, Shah R, Suelves AM, Foster CS: Road to remission: a comprehensive review of therapy in uveitis. Expert Opin Investig Drugs. 2011; 20(11):1497-515.

17. Kiss S, Ahmed M, Letko E, Foster CS. Long-term follow-up of patients with birdshot retinochoroidopathy treated with corticosteroid-sparing systemic immunomodulatory therapy. *Ophthalmology*. 2005;112(6):1066-1071.
18. Cervantes-Castaneda RA, Bhat P, Fortuna E, Acevedo S, Foster CS. Induction of durable remission in ocular inflammatory diseases. Eur J Ophthalmol. 2009: 19(1):118-23.
19. Forooghian F, Gulati N, Jabs DA. Restoration of retinal architecture following systemic immunosuppression in birdshot retinochoroidopathy. Ocul Immunol Inflamm. 2010 Dec;18(6):470-1.
20. Jabs DA, Rosenbaum JT, Foster CS, et al. Guidelines for the use of immunosuppressive drugs in patients with ocular inflammatory disorders. Am J Ophthalmol 2000;130:492–513.
21. Durrani K, Zakka FR, MD, Ahmed M et al. Systemic Therapy With Conventional and Novel Immunomodulatory Agents for Ocular Inflammatory Disease. Surv Ophthalmol 2011; 56(6):474—510.
22. Cervantes-Castañeda RA, Gonzalez-Gonzalez LA, Cordero-Coma M, Yilmaz T, Foster CS. Combined therapy of cyclosporine A and mycophenolate mofetil for the treatment of birdshotretinochoroidopathy: a 12-month follow-up.Br J Ophthalmol. 2013;97(5):637-43.
23. Quillen DA, Davis JB, Gottlieb JL, et al. The white dot syndromes. Am J Ophthalmol 2004;137:538 –50.
24. Priem HA, De Rouck A, De Laey JJ, Bird AC. Electrophysiologic studies in birdshot retinochoroidopathy. Am J Ophthalmol 1988;106:430–436.

25. Levinson RD, Gonzales CR. Birdshot retinochoroidopathy: immunopathogenesis, evaluation, and treatment. Ophthalmol Clin North Am 2002;15:343–50.
26. Monnet D, Brézin AP, Holland GN et al. Longitudinal cohort study of patients with birdshot retinochoroidopathy. I.Baseline clinical characteristics. Am J Ophthalmol. 2006 Jan;141(1):135-42.
27. de Courten C, Herbort CP. Potential role of computerized visual field testing for the appraisal and follow-up of birdshot retinochoroidopathy. Arch Ophthalmol 1998;116:1389 –1391.
28. Keane PA, Allie M, Turner SJ et al. Characterization of birdshot retinochoroidopathy using extramacular enhanced depth optical coherence tomography. JAMA Ophthalmol. 2013;131(3):341-50.
29. Witkin AJ, Duker JS, Ko TH, Fujimoto JG, Schuman JS. Ultrahigh resolution optical coherence tomography of birdshot retinochoroidopathy. Br J Ophthalmol. 2005;89(12):1660-1661.

Chapter 10

Biologic Response Modifier Therapy

Antoine P. Brézin

Until biologic response modifier therapy became available, treatment options for patients with birdshot retinochoroidopathy (BSRC) were limited to corticosteroids or immunosuppressants and, most frequently, a combination of both. Because birdshot retinochoroidopathy is a chronic disease, the duration of the treatment is usually longer than a year and adapted to its effect on inflammatory signs, such as vascular leakage and macular edema. The benefits of treatment are concomitantly judged on functional parameters such as visual acuity and visual fields. No randomized trials are available to guide therapeutic decisions. Infliximab has been the monoclonal antibody used for the largest number of patients with BSRC treated with a biologic response modifier. Small case-series or single case-reports have described favorable effects of tocilizumab, rituximab and daclizumab. Interferon-alpha and intravenous immunoglobulin have also been used. Adalimumab and gevokizumab are currently assessed in ongoing large-scale multicentric randomized treatment trials focused on intermediate or posterior uveitis allowing the inclusion of patients with birdshot retinochoroidopathy.

Biological Response Modifiers in BSRC

Biological response modifiers (BRM's) target specific molecules or pathways involved in inflammatory processes. BRM's include monoclonal antibodies, recombinant constructs, such as receptor constructs, as well as cytokines. An internationally accepted nomenclature is used in the naming of monoclonal antibodies (Table 1). Interferons and immunoglobulins are also usually counted among biological response modifiers. All are large molecules that can be currently administered only intravenously or subcutaneously. Biological response modifiers were first used in inflammatory rheumatic diseases such as rheumatoid arthritis. Their use has now spread to severe cases of uveitis, where several case-series have suggested efficacy.[1]
However, pending the results of ongoing large-scale randomized controlled trials, there are no established guidelines regarding their use in patients with chronic inflammatory eye diseases yet. As a model of autoimmune chronic

Table 1

Prefix	Target: Immune system	Source	Code	Suffix
Variable	**LI**	Human	**H**	**MAB**
		Humanized	**ZU**	
		Chimeric (Human/Foreign)	**XI**	
		Mouse	**O**	

uveitis, which can cause severe visual impairment, birdshot retinochoroidopathy is one of the causes of uveitis for which several biological response modifiers are thought to have a significant potential. Table 2 recapitulates published articles reporting the use of biological response modifiers in patients with birdshot retinochoroidopathy.

Table 2. Literature review regarding patients with birdshot chorioretinopathy treated by biological response modifiers

Name of Drug	*Mode of Action*	*Total Number of Patients*	*Patients with BSRC*	*Authors*	*Year Published*
Infliximab Remicade®	chimeric murine-human anti-TNF-alpha	22	22	Artornsombudh et al.	2013
Tocilizumab Actemra®	IL6 receptor blocker	5	3	Adán et al.	2013
Rituximab Rituxan®, MabThera®	Chimeric anti-CD20 (B-cell depletion)	1	1	Tomkins-Netzer	2013
Interferon alpha	Interferon alpha	6	2	Paire et al.	2010
Daclizumab Zenapax®	Humanized anti-IL-2 receptor (anti-CD25)	5	2	Yeh et al.	2008
Immunoglobulins	Intravenous immunoglobulin	37	37	Cassoux et al.	2002

Infliximab

Infliximab is a chimeric monoclonal antibody composed of the variable regions of murine antibody joined to the constant region of human immunoglobulin G1. The antibody binds with high affinity to both soluble and transmembrane forms of tumor necrosis factor alpha (TNF-α). Its route of administration is by intravenous infusion and the usual dose is 3–5 mg/kg body weight repeated after 2 and then every 4 to 8 weeks. Side-effects during infusion include dizziness and headaches, severe but rare reactions have also been reported. The strong immunosuppression induced by infliximab inhibits defense of infections. Latent tuberculosis is of particular concern and must be excluded by thoracic imaging, tuberculin skin testing and/or Quantiferon® test. Serology for viral hepatitis B and C and HIV are also required pretreatment tests.

Artornsombudh et al. have reported the effects of infliximab in a retrospective series of 22 patients (44 eyes) with birdshot retinochoroidopathy.[2] All patients were refractory to traditional immunosuppressive therapy. Control of inflammation was achieved in 81.82% of the patients at 6 months and in 88.9% of patients at 1 year.

Other monoclonal antibodies

Only a small number of patients with birdshot retinochoroidopathy have been treated by mononoclonal antibodies other than infliximab.

The use of tocilizumab, a fully humanized antibody that binds both to soluble and membrane bound IL-6 receptors, has been reported in five patients with refractory uveitic cystoid macular edema, of which three had birdshot retinochoroidopathy.[3] The treatment was successful to diminish the macular thickness, from a mean of 602 ± 236 µm at baseline, to 294.5 ± 94.5 µm at month 6. The median best-corrected visual acuity improved from 0.66±0.57 at baseline to 0.47 ± 0.62 at month 6 and sustained uveitis remission was achieved in all patients.

The use of rituximab, a chimeric (murine and human) monoclonal antibody directed against the CD20 antigen, has been reported in a single patient with refractory birdshot retinochoroidopathy.[4] Rituximab acts by targeting mature B lymphocytes and results in peripheral B cell depletion. Birdshot retinochoroidopathy is believed to be a disease involving T lymphocytes. However, the single case-report described a favorable effect of rituximab in a patient who was concomitantly treated by mycophenolate mofetil and whose dose of prednisolone was reduced to 5mg/day.

The use of daclizumab, a humanized anti-IL-2 receptor alpha antibody, has been reported in five patients with non-infectious uveitis, of whom two had birdshot retinochoroidopathy.[5] Patients demonstrated a decrease in vitreous haze and measures of intraocular inflammation after a one-year follow-up.

Interferon-alpha

Interferons are cytokines produced by dendritic plasmacytoid cells, but also by lymphocytes, macrophages, monocytes and glial cells. Interferon-alpha has antiviral, antiproliferative and immunomodulating effects. Six patients with uveitic macular edema, of whom two had birdshot retinochoroidopathy, were treated by interferon alpha.[6] A decrease in vitreous haze and measures of intraocular inflammation at final follow-up was reported. In this small case-series, a 189 ± 67 µm in macular thickness and an improvement of visual acuity of 0.35 ± 0.21 logMAR was observed.

Intravenous immunoglobulin

Intravenous immunoglobulin (IVIg) has been used for the treatment of several auto-immune diseases and particularly in idiopathic immune thrombocytopenia.

In a series of eighteen patients with birdshot retinochoroidopathy who were treated by IVIg and prospectively followed, inflammation improved on fluorescein angiography in 81% of the cases and cystoid macular edema decreased in 65% of the cases.[7]

Ongoing trials

As of September 1st, 2013, a number of clinical trials using biological agents are available to patients with birdshot retinochoroidopathy (ClinicalTrials.gov and Table 3). However, because of the rarity of the disease, none of these trials is focused specifically on patients with birdshot retinochoroidopathy. Inclusion criteria encompass patients with intermediate, posterior or panuveitis. Some trials are still in phase I-II and target a handful of patients. Only two biological agents, adalimumab and gevokizumab are currently under trial in large multicenter, randomized, controlled, double-masked, studies. For both of these agents, one trial is focused on patients with active inflammation, while the other targets patients who have controlled inflammation under their current treatment and who are switched to the study drug. Recruitment for both of these trials remains active and completion times are scheduled in 2015-2016, with results available approximately one to two years later.

Table 3.

Name of Drug	*Mode of action*	*Trial characteristics*	*Study identifier Estimated completion date*	*Number of centers; Planned number of patients*	*Population*	*Outcome measures*
Ustekinumab Stelara®	Human IL-12 and -23 antagonist	Phase 1-2 Safety/Efficacy Study Single Group Open Label	NCT01647152 June 2014	Single center 5 patients	Active int., post., and panuveitis	Safety Response to treatment
Tocilizumab Actemra®	IL6 receptor blocker	Phase 1-2 Randomized Parallel Assignment Single Blind	NCT01717170 (STOP-UVEITIS Study) Not yet recruiting	Single center 36 patients	Active int., post., and panuveitis	Safety Decrease of ≥ 2 steps in vitreous haze or resolution of haze
Adalimumab Humira®	Human anti-TNF	Phase 3 Randomized	NCT01138657 (Visual I) October 2014	Multicenter 250 patients	Active int., post., and panuveitis	Time to treatment failure after corticosteroids taper
Adalimumab Humira®	Human anti-TNF	Phase 3	NCT01124838 (Visual II) October 2014	Multicenter 250 patients	Inactive int., post., and panuveitis	Time to treatment failure after corticosteroids taper
Gevokizumab Xoma052	Humanized anti-IL1ß	Phase 3 Randomized Double Blind	NCT01684345 EYEGUARD™-A September 2015	Multicenter 300 patients	Active int., post., and panuveitis	Proportion of responders
Gevokizumab Xoma052	Humanized anti-IL1ß	Phase 3 Randomized Double Blind	NCT01747538 EYEGUARD™-C December 2014	Multicenter 300 patients	Controlled int., post., or pan- uveitis	Occurrence of uveitic disease
Secukinumab (AIN457)	Human anti-IL-17A	Phase 2-3 *Withdrawn*	NCT01327664 *Withdrawn*	Multicenter		
Basiliximab Simulect®	Chimeric mouse-human anti - α chain (CD25) of the IL-2 receptor of T cells	Phase 2 Randomized Double Blind	NCT00646425 November 2008	Multicenter 5 patients	Int., post., and panuveitis	Disease activity while tapering of concomitant immunosuppressive meds
Topical Interferon Gamma-1b Actimmune®	Interferon Gamma-1b	Phase 1-2 Single Group Open Label	NCT01376362 March 2012	Single center 5 patients	Cystoid macular edema secondary to uveitis	Macular thickening measured by OCT

Current questions on the use of biological response modifiers in BSRC

The data regarding the use of biological response modifiers in patients with birdshot retinochoroidopathy remain too limited to justify any of these treatment modalities as first line therapy. However, at least for infliximab, the current data suggest that this is a possible alternative to the classical treatment by immunosuppressants and corticosteroids in patients with refractory birdshot retinochoroidopathy. Whether biological response modifiers should best be used in addition to immunosuppressants or as stand-alone therapy remains an unanswered question.

Based on data stemming from the use of biological response modifiers in other auto-immune diseases, it is possible that these drugs have only a suspensive effect and that the inflammation will recur as the treatment is discontinued. Whether the long-term risk of recurrence differs between immunosuppressant-treated patients and those receiving biological response modifiers remains unanswered.

The costs of biological response modifiers are usually much greater than conventional therapies, which in most countries will impact decisions regarding which patients may be eligible for these treatments.

The short-term side-effects of the most common biological response modifiers are now well known. They include anaphylactoid type reactions such as fever, chills, headache, dyspnea or chest pain during infusions or shortly after. Infections are a major concern as biological response modifiers block one of the main pathways used in the defense against microbes. Tuberculosis is of particular concern and should be ruled out by systematic screening before the onset of treatment. Infections of the upper respiratory and urinary tracts, sepsis, several opportunistic infections and hepatitis B virus reactivation have all been reported. Drug-induced lupus and demyelinating disease are also a concern. Finally, the rate of cancers and lymphomas in patients treated by biological response modifiers might be increased. As biological response modifiers are rather new drugs, no patients have yet been treated for a decade or more, and some long-term side-effects may still remain to be recognized.[8] However, as with corticosteroids or classical immunosuppressants which both have known adverse effects, side-effects have to be balanced with the benefits of treatment.

References

1. Saadoun D, Bodaghi B, Bienvenu B, Wechsler B, Sene D, Trad S, Abad S, Cacoub P, Kodjikian L, Sève P.Biotherapies in inflammatory ocular disorders: Interferons, immunoglobulins, monoclonal antibodies. Autoimmun Rev. 2013;12:774-83.
2. Artornsombudh P, Gevorgyan O, Payal A, Siddique SS, Foster CS. Infliximab treatment of patients with birdshot retinochoroidopathy. Ophthalmology. 2013;120:588-92.
3. Adán A, Mesquida M, Llorenç V, Espinosa G, Molins B, Hernández MV, Pelegrín L. Tocilizumab treatment for refractory uveitis-related cystoid macular edema. Graefes Arch Clin Exp Ophthalmol. 2013 Jul 27.
4. Tomkins-Netzer O, Taylor SR, Lightman S. Can rituximab induce long-term disease remission in patients with intra-ocular non-infectious inflammation? Ophthalmologica. 2013;230:109-15.
5. Yeh S, Wroblewski K, Buggage R, Li Z, Kurup SK, Sen HN, Dahr S, Sran P, Reed GF, Robinson R, Ragheb JA, Waldmann TA, Nussenblatt RB. High-dose humanized anti-IL-2 receptor alpha antibody (daclizumab) for the treatment of active, non-infectious uveitis. J Autoimmun. 2008;31:91-7.
6. Paire V, Lebreton O, Weber M. Effectiveness of interferon alpha in the treatment of uveitis macular edema refractory to corticosteroid and/or immunosuppressive treatment. J Fr Ophtalmol. 2010;33:152-62.
7. Cassoux N, Goichot-Bonnat L, Karmochkine M, Georges F, Kullmann N, Lehoang P, Kazatchkine M. Efficacy of intravenous immunoglobulin in the treatment of Birdshot retinochoroidopathy. J Fr Ophtalmol. 2002;25:23-30.

8. Heiligenhaus A, Thurau S, Hennig M, Grajewski RS, Wildner G. Anti-inflammatory treatment of uveitis with biologicals: new treatment options that reflect pathogenetic knowledge of the disease. Graefes Arch Clin Exp Ophthalmol. 2010;248:1531-51.

Chapter 11

Corticosteroid Implant Therapy

Henry J. Kaplan, Niloofar Piri

Birdshot retinochoroidopathy is an intraocular inflammatory disease involving the posterior segment that can progress with the retention of good central visual acuity until there has been very substantial retinal damage and other functional visual loss. Monitoring of BSRC patients with BSRC every six months is therefore necessary to identify when aggressive medical therapy should be initiated. Since the inner and outer retinopathy of BSRC appear to involve both autoinflammation and autoimmunity combined treatment with both corticosteroids, as well as immunomodulatory therapy (IMT), will need to be employed in most patients.

Treatment for intraocular inflammation should be based on an understanding of the immune pathogenesis of the disease. Therefore, we will first discuss the components of immunity that are recognized for birdshot retinochoroidopathy (BSRC) – namely, autoinflammation and autoimmunity.[1] We then will discuss the treatment paradigm that is most frequently used by other uveitis specialists, as well as that which is used at the University of Louisville. We will talk about corticosteroid therapy and the transition to immunomodulatory therapy.

The immunopathogenesis of BSRC appears to involve both autoinflammation and autoimmunity. Autoinflammation is a dysregulation of innate immunity, the limb of the immune response that provides an immediate host immune response to infectious agents via receptors that recognize microbial-specific molecular patterns (pathogen-associated molecular patterns, PAMPS).

There are many different PAMP receptors and they are located on the plasma cell membrane or intracellular compartments. For example, toll like receptors (TLRs) are located on plasma membranes and endosomes; C-type lectins (CTLs) on plasma membranes; retinoic acid-inducible gene (RIG-1)-like helicase within the cytoplasm; NOD-like receptors (NLRs) within the cytoplasm.

The pro-inflammatory cascade of innate immunity involves PAMPS, danger-associated molecular patterns (DAMPS), and the inflammasome. The latter is an intracellular protein complex that is activated by numerous danger signals including PAMPS and DAMPS. Activation of the inflammasome leads to the cleavage and activation of caspase-1 and subsequent cleavage of pro-IL-1β to its mature, active form, which is then released from the cell. Once released, IL-1β binds to the IL-1R, leading to downstream signaling and a cascade of inflammation involving other pro-inflammatory cytokines (e.g. TNFa).

An interesting insight into the immunopathogenesis of BSRC can be obtained from an analysis of clinical reports in the literature, as well as anecdotal experience. Sorbin et al[2] reported the outcome of daclizumab in the treatment of BSRC refractory to IMT. Over a mean follow-up of 25.6

months, seven of eight patients had either stabilization or improvement of visual acuity in both eyes and complete resolution of vitreous inflammation. However, the ERG parameters continued to decline in five of eight patients despite adequate inflammatory control – recognized by an increase in implicit time of the 30Hz flicker response in the full field ERG. A more recent study by Atornsombudh[3] reported the outcome of infliximab treatment for BSRC refractory to conventional IMT. After initiating infliximab, control of inflammation (vitritis, retinal vasculitis, and cystoid macular edema [CME]) was achieved in 81.8% at six months and in 88.9% at one year follow-up. The rate of CME decreased from 22.7% at baseline to 6.7% at one year after starting treatment. However, progression of the disease was characterized by loss of visual field and changes in electrophysiology. Although the authors did not mention that the implicit time of the 30Hz flicker ERG was prolonged, they did state that it was performed semiannually. Presumably, this was the criterion that they used on electrophysiology to conclude that progression of the disease had continued with loss of visual field.

We have hypothesized from these studies, as well as our understanding of the immune response, that HLA-A2902 antigen presenting cells (e.g. dendritic cells) from BSRC patients are hyper-responsive in two ways: (1) in response to PAMPS/DAMPS which enhances innate immunity, and (2) in antigen presentation, which enhances adaptive immunity. Since HLA-A29 is a class I MHC molecule the A-29 motif should present antigen to CD8+ but not CD4+ T-cells. We believe that activated CD8+ cytotoxic T lymphocytes are responsible for BSRC lesions (i.e. outer retinopathy), the reason that IMT can inhibit the progression of photoreceptor death. Additionally, innate immunity (i.e. cytokines/ILs) is responsible for vitritis, retinal vasculitis, and CME (i.e. inner retinopathy), the reason biologic therapy is needed to inhibit inner retinopathy. Thus, both immune suppression and biologic therapy may be needed in patients with BSRC to achieve complete quiescence and why high dose corticosteroid therapy is required to inhibit both inner and outer retinopathy.

The retina and choroid seem independently involved in the inflammatory process. The innate immune response is presumably associated with vitreoretinal features like vitritis, CME, and retinal vasculitis; the adaptive immune response with retinochoroidopathy, i.e. the characteristic chorioretinal lesions that progress, resulting in permanent vision loss from photoreceptor damage. Our therapeutic approach is guided by the belief that the innate immune response is effectively controlled by corticosteroids and biologics, while the adaptive immune response is more effectively controlled by immune suppression. Thus, the current approach to treatment by most uveitis specialists involves the use of corticosteroids as the first therapeutic option – either alone or concomitant with IMT. Oral corticosteroids or intravitreal corticosteroids are generally used since the disease is bilateral. The latter would include the intravitreal injection of Kenalog (4mg/0.1cc) or the insertion of corticosteroid slow-release devices such as Retisert or Ozurdex. Although both devices are FDA approved, there are several other intravitreal devices that are under development for the delivery of corticosteroids – e.g., I-vation™TA, a triamcinolone acetonide metal-coiled implant; Iluvien™, a non-biodegradable implant.

Retisert is a non-biodegradable intravitreal implant of flucinolone acetonide. It is FDA approved for the treatment of chronic and infectious uveitis infecting the posterior segment. It consists of a 1.5mm tablet coated with polyvinyl alcohol and silicone laminate. It measures 3mm x 2mm x 6mm and has an initial release rate of 0.6μg per day, which after the first month decreases to a steady rate of 0.3 to 0.4μg per day over approximately 30 months. In the treatment of corticosteroid responsive uveitis, Retisert significantly reduced uveitis recurrences, decreased the need for adjunctive therapy and 25% of implanted eyes had a 3-line or greater increase in visual acuity at 34 weeks. Unfortunately, significant problems associated with this implant at 24 months involved the development of a cataract which required surgery in 89.4%, as well as glaucoma requiring surgery in 30.6%. Additionally, insertion of the implant requires an operating room and the implant is non-biodegradable. The MUST research group did a randomized comparison of systemic corticosteroid therapy with immune suppression versus Retisert.[4] They noted no advantage to either treatment regimen, and thus, recommended that individualized patient treatment should be exercised.

In contrast, Ozurdex is a biodegradable implant that delivers dexamethasone. It is also FDA approved and administered via a 22 gauge applicator. The medication is delivered within a PLGA polymer matrix and releases 0.7mg of dexamethasone over six months. The PLGA matrix fully degrades to lactic acid and glycolic acid enabling extended release over a six month period. Ozurdex was investigated by the HURON study group.[5] Both the 0.35mg and 0.7mg dexamethasone implant was associated with less intraocular inflammation in non-infectious posterior uveitis. Visual acuity was improved at six months versus a sham procedure. Unfortunately, no comparative effectiveness trial was conducted using either intravitreal Kenalog or Retisert. With the Ozurdex implant an intraocular pressure peak greater than 25mmHg was higher for the implant versus sham (8.7/7.1 versus 4.2%). It was concluded that the dexamethasone implant may be used safely and effectively for the treatment of intermediate and posterior uveitis. Efficacy in the treatment of central retinal vein occlusion was also noted in subsequent studies although again there was no comparison to the effectiveness of treatment with other standard therapeutic protocols.

There is only one publication in the literature which looked at the outcome of treatment of BSRC with an intravitreal sustained-release flucinolone acetonide-containing device (i.e. Retisert)[6]. In a retrospective case study, the medical records of 22 patients were reviewed. Treatment with Retisert was initiated depending on clinical assessment of the degree of intraocular inflammation, the response to prior treatment, and the patient's preference. The authors concluded that CME, vitritis, and retinal vasculitis were well-controlled. However, the results of electrophysiology and visual fields were not analyzed due to a wide variation among the patients. Thus, the true clinical effectiveness of Retisert for BSRC was not established. There are two other reports in the literature describing treatment of BSRC with

Retisert but they are simply clinical observations involving one or two patients.[7,8]

Our approach at UofL involves the use of oral prednisone (0.75-1.0 mg/ kg, in divided doses) for the initial control of vitritis, CME and retinal vasculitis for the first two weeks, and then tapered over the next 2-3 months. If the patient is intolerant of systemic corticosteroids or noncompliant, an intravitreal injection of Kenalog or insertion of the Ozurdex implant is performed. Our preference is for the use of intravitreal Kenalog because of the dramatically lower cost. IMT is started with objective evidence of retinal damage (i.e. prolonged implicit time with the 30Hz cone flicker response, abnormal automated Humphrey visual field 30-2 or decreased dark adaptation) either at the time of the initial office visit or upon subsequent presentation. These tests are performed every six months. We would start IMT when initially seeing the patient if there was evidence of documented retinal abnormality on any of these tests on the first visit after consultation with the patient.

References

1. Doria A, Zen M, Bettio S, et al. Autoinflammation and autoimmunity: bridging the divide. Autoimmun Rev. 2012:12(1):22-30.
2. Sorbin L, Huang JJ, Christen W, et al. Daclizumab for treatment of birdshot retinochoroidopathy. *Arch Ophthalmol.* 2008:126(2):186-91.
3. Artornsombudh P, Gevorgyan O, Payal A. Infliximab treatment of patients with birdshot retinochoroidopathy. *Ophthalmology.* 2013:120(3):588-92.
4. MUST Research Group. Randomized comparison of systemic therapy (systemic corticosteroids + immune suppression) vs Retisert. Ophthalmol. 2011:118(10):1916-26.
5. Ozurdex HURON Study Group. Dexamethasone intravitreal implant for non-infectious posterior uveitis. *Arch Ophthalmol.* 2011(5):545-53.
6. Rush RB, Goldstein DA, Callanan DG, et al. Outcomes of birdshot retinochoroidopathy treated with an intravitreal sustained-release fluocinolone acetonide-containing device. *Am J Ophthalmol.* 2011:151(4):630-6.
7. Kisma N, Robson AG, Graham E. Long term outcome of birdshot retinochoroidopathy treated by Fluocinolone Acetonide Intravitreal Implant (Retisert): A case series report. *ARVO Abstract.* 2011.
8. Terrada C, Bruneau S, Perrenoud F, et al. Role of intravitreal dexamethasone implant in the treatment of birdshot retinochoroidopathy. *J Fr Ophtalmol.* 2011:35(9):745-8.

Chapter 12

New Therapeutic Strategies in Development

Bahram Bodaghi

Treatment modalities of Birdshot retinochoroidopathy (BSRC) have dramatically improved the visual outcome of the patients during the last decade. However, severe cases and those resisting to conventional immunomodulatory agents encouraged the development of new strategies. Different options including new generation of immunosuppressors and pro-inflammatory cytokines inhibitors are currently available. Interleukin-17, IL-6 and IL-1 blockers are potential candidates if intraocular levels of these inflammatory markers are considered. Controlled clinical trials are required in order to evaluate their efficacy, even though the lack of optimal endpoints may be difficult to overcome, leading to study failure. Safety issues need also to be addressed with newer drugs or routes of administration. Immune tolerance may be obtained with cell therapy, especially polyclonal regulatory T lymphocytes, administered intravitreally after in vitro activation. Future therapy will need an optimal understanding of BSRC pathogenesis and better delivery systems in order to propose a personalized strategy with minimal side effects.

Introduction

Birdshot retinochoroidopathy is one of the most emblematic uveitic entities. With a very-well defined genetic background associated with the analysis of an appropriate animal model and studies on pathogenesis, it seems easy to propose an efficient therapeutic strategy in order to achieve long-term quiescence and maintain vision. It is now widely admitted that treatment is mandatory and should be initiated early during the course of the disease. Long-term delay may lead to permanent visual loss and severe handicap. However, in the absence of controlled clinical trials, the optimal approach remains controversial. Some schools of thought propose local therapy for this typically ocular inflammation, without predominant extraocular autoimmune disorders, whereas others recommend systemic therapy, controlling the immune network. High dose cyclosporine A, proposed in the 1980s was efficient but induced irreversible renal toxicity.[1] Systemic or intravitreal corticosteroids associated with conventional immunosuppressors represent the first line of therapy. Resistant cases and poor tolerance have encouraged the development of more targeted strategies. Developing new therapeutic tools must consider different major issues such as effectiveness, reduced toxicity, rescue of refractory cases, corticosteroids-sparing ability.[2,3] The future depends on new pharmacological compounds, new routes of administration as well as cell therapy.

Pathogenesis

Development of new therapeutic alternatives strongly relies on the understanding of BSRC pathophysiology. More than all other autoimmune uveitic entities, animal models and human studies have added crucial informations that must be taken into consideration before any further progress.

Experimental models

Different animal models of uveitis developed in mice, rats, guinea pigs or primates may be transposed to BSRC. However, HLA-A29 is associated with BSRC in more than 95% of cases, thus representing the strongest link between an HLA antigen and a human disease. Despite this important finding, the pathogenesis of BSRC remains poorly understood. HLA-A29-transgenic mice develop a spontaneous disease characterized by retinal vasculopathy and papillitis with inflammatory lesions in the choroid and the retina leading to photoreceptor alterations.[4,5]

Human pathology

Pathology features of a patient from the University of California, San Francisco, disclosed lesions similar to those described initially by Steve Ryan including staining of vessel walls and collection of lymphocytes around choroidal vessels. Both retina and choroid are involved in birdshot retinochoroidopathy. In the case reported by Rao et al. uveitis is mainly a nongranulomatous chronic inflammation with presence of CD8+ T cells and modified histiocytes (CD68+). In birdshot retinochoroidopathy, there is preservation of the inner and outer choroid from the lymphocytic infiltration. Depending on the disease stage, the cellular infiltrate may include more CD4+ or CD8+ cells. Therefore, therapeutic strategy may depend on the disease stage.

Immune mediators in patients with BSRC

More recently, Kuiper et al. reported on the level of 23 immune mediators in paired aqueous humor and serum of 16 patients with HLA-A29-associated birdshot retinochoroidopathy.[6] Interestingly, the ocular levels of IL-2, IL-17, IL-1b, IL-6 and TNF-α were elevated compared with that of controls. Moreover, a significant positive correlation was noted between IL-17 and both IL-2 and IL-23, but also between IL-2 and IL-23. These findings are important to consider for selection of new biologic agents and development of new clinical trials in patients with BSRC.

Drugs in development

During the last 10 years, an increasing number of drugs have been evaluated in clinical trials, including patients with BSRC. Vitreous haze is currently the main endpoint used for efficacy evaluation but it is not the best activity marker in this group of patients. Therefore, composite endpoints, including visual acuity and macular edema, may be more appropriate to consider in the future.

Revisiting Conventional immunosuppressors

New generation of Calcineurin inhibitors

Voclosporin (E-ISA247) originates from a modification on the first amino acid residue of the cyclosporine A (CsA) molecule.[7,8] It inhibits T cell activation[9] and in vitro studies have shown that voclosporin is approximately four times more potent than CsA with a better safety profile due to the use of lower doses. The drug is currently used for the prevention of organ transplant rejection and treatment of psoriasis. The LUMINATE (LX211 Uveitis Multicentre Investigation of a New Approach to TrEatment) studies were designed to evaluate the efficacy and safety of Voclosporin in 3 placebo-controlled, dose-ranging, randomized trials.[10] For the first time, two groups were defined based on disease activity (LUMINATE Active and LUMINATE Maintenance). The third trial was dedicated to anterior uveitis. The studies compared 0.2, 0.4 and 0.6 mg/kg b.i.d. with placebo in patients with different types of uveitis. In the study on active uveitis (LX211-01), voclosporin has demonstrated efficacy with reduction of vitreous haze (50% in the 0.4 mg/kg b.i.d. group compared with 29% in the placebo recipients). In the study on controlled uveitis (LX211-02), voclosporin at 0.4 mg/kg b.i.d. reduced the rate of inflammatory relapses by 50% at the 26-week primary endpoint compared with the placebo group. Systemic IMT were used in nearly 90% of patients in this group prior to randomization and were discontinued before inclusion. In the last trial (LX211-03) on anterior uveitis, all patients experienced improvement. Hypertension, diarrhea and decreased renal function were the most common adverse events reported with voclosporin (rates superior to 5% and higher than placebo).

Due to a unique significant trial (LX211-01), a second phase 3-study for active non-infectious intermediate, posterior, and panuveitis was initiated in order to obtain registration for its use and application in uveitis. Results were analyzed in 2012 and showed no difference between the 0.4 mg/kg b.i.d. group and placebo. This finding was surprising regarding the use of CsA for many years in patients with uveitis, especially those with BSRC. Overestimation of vitreous haze at inclusion may explain part of these controversial results and highlights the limitations of this endpoint.

Sirolimus

Rapamycin is a natural antibiotic identified from Streptomyces hygroscopicus, in the 1970s.[11] This macrolide has been approved for the prevention of solid organ transplant rejection. Rapamycin inhibits the actions of a multifunctional serine-threonine kinase (mTOR). Inhibition of the latter results in G1 cell cycle arrest blocking the cell cycle from G1 to S phase in various cell types, including T and B lymphocytes.[12] Rapamycin may also negatively modulate VEGF transcription as well as other pro-angiogenic factors. The systemic use of sirolimus showed efficacy but also intolerable side effects.[13] Both subconjunctival[14] and intravitreal routes of administration have been developed. The SAVE study, a phase I randomized open-label trial (Sirolimus as a Therapeutic Approach for Noninfectious Uveitis) has been performed in the US to evaluate the efficacy and safety of intravitreal or subconjunctival sirolimus in 30 patients with noninfectious posterior, intermediate, and panuveitis.[15] At the primary endpoint (6 months) both routes of administration were able to induce total or partial control of uveitis activity and to reduce recurrences. Injections were safe and leaded to phase III multicenter randomized trials in order to confirm the preliminary data on efficacy and safety. This strategy is interesting to consider as it may avoid systemic side effects of sirolimus and those of intravitreal corticosteroids.

New Generation of Biologic agents

TNF alpha inhibitors and alpha interferon have been used with interesting results in severe cases of BSRC.[16,17] However, efficacy may be limited over time and side effects are important to consider in some cases. Based on cytokines analysis, other biologics may be proposed in the future.

Inhibitors of IL-6

IL-6 has been frequently associated with noninfectious uveitis based on intraocular assessment of cytokines.[18] It is produced by T cells, monocytes and macrophages. It plays a major role in the maturation of B cells into Ig-secreting cells but also differentiation of Th17 lymphocytes. Inhibition of IL-6 seems to suppress EAU via inhibition of Th17 cells.[19,20] Interestingly, IL-6 can promote IL-17 production by natural killer cells. Natural killer cells and some T cells have HLA class I-specific killer immunoglobulin-like receptors, which regulate the activity of these cells. Combinations of killer immunoglobulin-like receptor–HLA-A29 gene variations have been proposed to increase susceptibility of developing BSRC.[21]

Tocilizumab (ACTEMRA/RoACTEMRA) is a humanized IgG1 monoclonal antibody against both soluble and membrane-bound IL-6. The drug was approved in 2010 to treat refractory forms of rheumatoid arthritis. Systemic side-effects are important to consider with tocilizumab (hypertension, infections, gastrointestinal disorders, leukopenia, conjunctivitis and hypothyroidism). Authors have reported on the efficacy of tocilizumab in small case series of patients with severe uveitis.[22,23] Phase II trials are currently planned for systemic administration of new generations of anti-IL6 molecules in patients with noninfectious posterior uveitis.

Inhibitor of IL-17

Interleukin (IL)-17A, secreted by T-helper (Th)17 cells, is recognized as one of the main proinflammatory cytokines in immune-mediated inflammatory diseases.[24] It enhances T cell priming and stimulates the production of other proinflammatory molecules such as IL-1, IL-6, TNF-α, NOS-2 and chemokines resulting in inflammation.

Secukinumab is a selective, high-affinity, fully human monoclonal antibody that binds and neutralizes human IL-17A, potentially inhibiting the expression of other proinflammatory cytokines and effector proteins and preventing the activation of neutrophil granulocytes, macrophages, epithelial cells, and fibroblasts. Secukinumab has been evaluated in patients with Behçet's disease (BD) and those with noninfectious uveitis in three multicenter, randomized, double-masked, placebo-controlled, dose-ranging phase III studies: SHIELD (118 patients with BD), INSURE (31 patients with active noninfectious patients), and ENDURE (125 patients with quiescent noninfectious uveitis).[25] BD was excluded in INSURE and ENDURE trials. There were no statistically significant differences in uveitis recurrence between the secukinumab treatment groups and placebo groups in any of the 3 studies. However, secukinumab was associated with a significant reduction in mean total post-baseline immunosuppressive medication score ($P = 0.019$) in the SHIELD study. There was no loss in visual acuity reported in any treatment group during follow-up in all 3 studies. The frequencies of ocular and nonocular side effects seemed to be higher among secukinumab groups versus placebo across the 3 studies. The use of concomitant immunosuppressive therapy in all treatment groups at baseline and during the study may have played a role in the lack of significant difference between all groups on the primary efficacy end point of the SHIELD study. Moreover, the dynamics of IL-17 expression may be different among patients and explain the results.

Inhibitor of IL-23

Interleukin-23 (IL-23) is a heterodimeric cytokine consisting of two subunits: p40, which is also a component of the IL-12 cytokine, p19, which is considered the IL-23 alpha subunit. IL-23 is produced by dendritic cells and macrophages. It promotes upregulation of the matrix metalloprotease MMP9, increases angiogenesis and reduces CD8+ T-cell infiltration. It stimulates naïve CD4+ T cells to differentiate into Th17 cells.[26] Ustekinumab (STELARA, Centocor) is a human monoclonal antibody directed against IL-12 and IL-23 and used in patients with psoriasis.[27] It has been shown safe and effective in 2 phase III trials on moderate to severe psoriasis. There is an increased risk of infection associated with the drug.

Inhibitors of IL-1 (anakinra, rilonacept, canakinumab, gevokizumab)

IL-1 is a proinflammatory cytokine that plays a major role in chronic inflammation.[28] It may increase T helper cell costimulation, B cell proliferation and NK cell activation. This therapeutic strategy has previously shown efficacy in patients with auto-inflammatory conditions such as cryopirin-associated periodic syndromes (CAPS).

Anakinra is an interleukin-1 receptor antagonist. Its safety and efficacy have been analyzed in 3 randomized, double-masked, placebo-controlled trials of patients with rheumatoid arthritis. A study has shown the efficacy of anakinra in children with CINCA syndrome, including ocular inflammation.[29] However, other types of uveitis or ocular involvement have not been studied so far. Daily subcutaneous administration is one of the most important limitations of the drug.

Rilonacept consists of the extracellular domains of the Il-1-RAcP and the Il-1-R1 fused to the Fc portion of human

IgG1. It binds Il-1β and Il-1α with high affinity and is administered subcutaneously beginning with a loading dose followed by a weekly injection of half the loading dose. Canakinumab is a specific human monoclonal IgG1 antibody targeted against Il-1β. This antibody has no cross-reactivity with Il-1α or with the Il-1-R1 receptor. Canakinumab is also administered subcutaneously, but every 8 weeks.

These two drugs have not been evaluated in clinical trials for uveitis.

The most common side effects (>10% of treated patients) are reactions at the injection site, inflammation of the upper respiratory tract or sinuses and headache.

More recently, an open-label pilot study of gevokizumab (XOMA 052, humanized monoclonal antibody against IL-1β; XOMA LLC, Berkeley, CA) in the treatment of 7 patients with acute exacerbations of uveitis in Behçet's disease showed a rapid onset of effect and a sustained reduction in intraocular inflammation.[30] XOMA and SERVIER jointly develop an IL-1β targeted monoclonal antibody (gevokizumab) for the treatment of noninfectious intermediate, posterior and pan-uveitis, including BD. Gevokizumab (XOMA 052/S 78989) is a potent monoclonal antibody with unique allosteric modulating properties and the potential to treat patients with a wide variety of inflammatory diseases. Three clinical trials are currently designed in order to evaluate the efficacy and safety of gevokizumab in patients with Behçet's disease (Eyeguard B), active (Eyeguard A) or controlled (Eyeguard C) noninfectious posterior or panuveitis. Patients with BSRC may be included in both Eyeguard A and C depending on the level of inflammation.

New modalities of drug administration

Iontophoresis and nanoparticles for uveitis

Ionotophoresis is a noninvasive technique used to allow the penetration of drugs through ocular tissues with a low electric current. This strategy may be an alternative to intravitreal injections. However, controlled clinical trials are still missing and the procedure is not yet routinely available. Moreover, adverse events such as retinal or choroidal burns may be observed with high current densities and duration of the procedure. Studies have currently focused on anterior uveitis and efficacy has not been evaluated in patients with BSRC.

The use of nanoparticles is another procedure and has been reported in glaucoma, infectious and noninfectious uveitis. As mentioned for iontophoresis, trials evaluating the efficacy of nanoparticles have not been performed.

Cell therapy

Regulatory T cells play a major role in the modulation of the immune system. They are key players in the induction of immune tolerance. Naturally occurring thymus-derived CD4+CD25+ Tregs are a subset of T cells representing 5%-10% of the total peripheral CD4+ T cells. Alteration of

Tregs balance may lead to neoplasia or autoimmunity. Tregs are attractive tools for immunotherapeutic strategies. We have previously reported the efficacy and safety of specific or polyclonal CD4(+)CD25(+) regulatory T cells in a mice model of uveitis.[31] Based on promising results in this experimental model, a prospective clinical trial has been approved to evaluate the safety of intravitreal administration of autologous Tregs in patients with severe noninfectious uveitis. Inclusion of patients has been initiated and preliminary results are expected before the end of the year. BSRC may be a potential indication for this type of approach.

Conclusion

During the last ten years the field of uveitis has experienced the development of new generations of immunomodulatory drugs and biological agents. However, it is difficult to identify the most appropriate strategy in patients with BSRC, even though biomarker studies have facilitated our understanding of its pathogenesis. Results obtained in animal models and patients remain insufficient to identify the best drug or combination of molecules, which may be proposed to the patients. Further studies will allow clinicians to develop a personalized approach taking into account the control of intraocular inflammation but also neuroprotective options in order to avoid irreversible damages in patients with BSRC.

References

1. Tostivint I, du Montcel ST, Jaudon MC, et al. Renal outcome after ciclosporin-induced nephrotoxicity. Nephrol Dial Transplant. 2007;22(3):880-885. Epub 2006 Nov 2024.
2. Gomes Bittencourt M, Sepah YJ, Do DV, et al. New treatment options for noninfectious uveitis. In: Miserocchi E, Modorati G, Foster CS, eds. New Treatments in Noninfectious Uveitis. Basel: Karger; 2012:134-161.
3. Larson T, Nussenblatt RB, Sen HN. Emerging drugs for uveitis. Expert Opin Emerg Drugs. 2011;16(2):309-322. doi: 310.1517/14728214.14722011.14537824. Epub 14722011 Jan 14728216.
4. de Kozak Y, Camelo S, Pla M. Pathological aspects of spontaneous uveitis and retinopathy in HLA-A29 transgenic mice and in animal models of retinal autoimmunity: relevance to human pathologies. Ophthalmic Res. 2008;40(3-4):175-180. doi: 110.1159/000119872. Epub 000112008 Apr 000119818.
5. Szpak Y, Vieville JC, Tabary T, et al. Spontaneous retinopathy in HLA-A29 transgenic mice. Proc Natl Acad Sci U S A. 2001;98(5):2572-2576. Epub 2001 Feb 2513.
6. Kuiper JJ, Mutis T, de Jager W, de Groot-Mijnes JD, Rothova A. Intraocular interleukin-17 and proinflammatory cytokines in HLA-A29-associated birdshot retinochoroidopathy. Am J Ophthalmol. 2011;152(2):177-182.e171. doi: 110.1016/j.ajo.2011.1001.1031. Epub 2011 May 1013.

7. Anglade E, Aspeslet LJ, Weiss SL. A new agent for the treatment of noninfectious uveitis: rationale and design of three LUMINATE (Lux Uveitis Multicenter Investigation of a New Approach to Treatment) trials of steroid-sparing voclosporin. Clin Ophthalmol. 2008;2(4):693-702.
8. Anglade E, Yatscoff R, Foster R, Grau U. Next-generation calcineurin inhibitors for ophthalmic indications. Expert Opin Investig Drugs. 2007;16(10):1525-1540.
9. Cunningham MA, Austin BA, Li Z, et al. LX211 (voclosporin) suppresses experimental uveitis and inhibits human T cells. Invest Ophthalmol Vis Sci. 2009;50(1):249-255. doi: 210.1167/iovs.1108-1891. Epub 2008 Aug 1115.
10. Sepah YJ, Metcalf B, Khwaja A, et al. Voclosporin: a potentially promising therapeutic agent for noninfectious uveitis. Expert Rev Ophthalmol. 2011;6:281-286.
11. Pennesi G, Caspi RR. Genetic control of susceptibility in clinical and experimental uveitis. Int Rev Immunol. 2002;21(2-3):67-88.
12. Kahan BD, Podbielski J, Napoli KL, Katz SM, Meier-Kriesche HU, Van Buren CT. Immunosuppressive effects and safety of a sirolimus/cyclosporine combination regimen for renal transplantation. Transplantation. 1998;66(8):1040-1046.
13. Shanmuganathan VA, Casely EM, Raj D, et al. The efficacy of sirolimus in the treatment of patients with refractory uveitis. Br J Ophthalmol. 2005;89(6):666-669.

14. Sen HN, Larson TA, Meleth AD, Smith WM, Nussenblatt RB. Subconjunctival sirolimus for the treatment of chronic active anterior uveitis: results of a pilot trial. Am J Ophthalmol. 2012;153(6):1038-1042. doi: 1010.1016/j.ajo.2011.1012.1018. Epub 2012 Apr 1031.
15. NCT00908466., Cgi., http://clinicaltrialsgov/ct2/show/NCT00908466.
16. Artornsombudh P, Gevorgyan O, Payal A, Siddique SS, Foster CS. Infliximab treatment of patients with birdshot retinochoroidopathy. Ophthalmology. 2013;120(3):588-592. doi: 510.1016/j.ophtha.2012.1005.1048. Epub 2012 Nov 1021.
17. Saadoun D, Bodaghi B, Bienvenu B, et al. Biotherapies in inflammatory ocular disorders: Interferons, immunoglobulins, monoclonal antibodies. Autoimmun Rev. 2013;12(7):774-783. doi: 710.1016/j.autrev.2013.1002.1002. Epub 2013 Mar 1015.
18. Yoshimura T, Sonoda KH, Ohguro N, et al. Involvement of Th17 cells and the effect of anti-IL-6 therapy in auto-immune uveitis. Rheumatology (Oxford). 2009;48(4):347-354. doi: 310.1093/rheumatology/ken1489. Epub 2009 Jan 1022.
19. Haruta H, Ohguro N, Fujimoto M, et al. Blockade of interleukin-6 signaling suppresses not only th17 but also interphotoreceptor retinoid binding protein-specific Th1 by promoting regulatory T cells in experimental auto-immune uveoretinitis. Invest Ophthalmol Vis Sci. 2011;52(6):3264-3271. doi: 3210.1167/iovs.3210-6272.

20. Hohki S, Ohguro N, Haruta H, et al. Blockade of interleukin-6 signaling suppresses experimental autoimmune uveoretinitis by the inhibition of inflammatory Th17 responses. Exp Eye Res. 2010;91(2):162-170. doi: 110.1016/j.exer.2010.1004.1009. Epub 2010 Apr 1024.
21. Levinson RD, Du Z, Luo L, et al. Combination of KIR and HLA gene variants augments the risk of developing birdshot retinochoroidopathy in HLA-A*29-positive individuals. Genes Immun. 2008;9(3):249-258. doi: 210.1038/gene.2008.1013. Epub 2008 Mar 1013.
22. Adan A, Mesquida M, Llorenc V, et al. Tocilizumab treatment for refractory uveitis-related cystoid macular edema. Graefes Arch Clin Exp Ophthalmol. 2013;27:27.
23. Muselier A, Bielefeld P, Bidot S, Vinit J, Besancenot JF, Bron A. Efficacy of tocilizumab in two patients with anti-TNF-α refractory uveitis. Ocul Immunol Inflamm. 2011;19(5):382-383. doi: 310.3109/09273948.09272011.09606593.
24. Gu C, Wu L, Li X. IL-17 family: Cytokines, receptors and signaling. Cytokine. 2013;3(13):00638-00638.
25. Dick AD, Tugal-Tutkun I, Foster S, et al. Secukinumab in the treatment of noninfectious uveitis: results of three randomized, controlled clinical trials. Ophthalmology. 2013;120(4):777-787. doi: 710.1016/j.ophtha.2012.1009.1040. Epub 2013 Jan 1013.
26. Qu N, Xu M, Mizoguchi I, et al. Pivotal Roles of T-Helper 17-Related Cytokines, IL-17, IL-22, and IL-23, in Inflammatory Diseases. Clin Dev Immunol. 2013;2013:968549.(doi):10.1155/2013/968549. Epub 962013 Jul 968514.

27. McInnes IB, Kavanaugh A, Gottlieb AB, et al. Efficacy and safety of ustekinumab in patients with active psoriatic arthritis: 1 year results of the phase 3, multicentre, double-blind, placebo-controlled PSUMMIT 1 trial. Lancet. 2013;382(9894):780-789. doi: 710.1016/S0140-6736(1013)60594-60592. Epub 62013 Jun 60513.
28. Willermain F, Rosenbaum JT, Bodaghi B, et al. Interplay between innate and adaptive immunity in the development of non-infectious uveitis. Prog Retin Eye Res. 2012;31(2):182-194. doi: 110.1016/j.preteyeres.2011.1011.1004. Epub 2011 Nov 1022.
29. Neven B, Marvillet I, Terrada C, et al. Long-term efficacy of the interleukin-1 receptor antagonist anakinra in ten patients with neonatal-onset multisystem inflammatory disease/chronic infantile neurologic, cutaneous, articular syndrome. Arthritis Rheum. 2010;62(1):258-267. doi: 210.1002/art.25057.
30. Gul A, Tugal-Tutkun I, Dinarello CA, et al. Interleukin-1beta-regulating antibody XOMA 052 (gevokizumab) in the treatment of acute exacerbations of resistant uveitis of Behcet's disease: an open-label pilot study. Ann Rheum Dis. 2012;71(4):563-566. doi: 510.1136/annrheumdis-2011-155143. Epub 152011 Nov 155114.
31. Terrada C, Fisson S, De Kozak Y, et al. Regulatory T cells control uveoretinitis induced by pathogenic Th1 cells reacting to a specific retinal neoantigen. J Immunol. 2006;176(12):7171-7179.

Chapter 13

Identifying Gaps in Knowledge

Albert T. Vitale

Birdshot retinochoroidopathy (BSRC) is an uncommon but well characterized chronic, bilateral posterior uveitis which is uniquely associated with the human leukocyte antigen (HLA) – A29 phenotype. While autoimmune mechanisms are thought to play an important role in its pathogenesis, its etiology remains unknown. Important questions remain in our understanding of BSRC with respect to its pathogenesis, epidemiology, optimal treatment and prognosis including the determinants of remission and relapse, as well as the best strategy for monitoring disease activity, progression and response to therapy with electroretinographic and psychophysical testing, established and emerging imaging modalities, and peripheral cytokines profiles. The identification of these gaps in our knowledge of BSRC in the context our current understanding of this disease in each of these areas will illuminate fruitful avenues for future prospective investigation.

Introduction

Birdshot retinochoroidopathy (BSRC) is an uncommon but well characterized chronic, bilateral posterior uveitis occurring predominantly among middle aged, Caucasian patients of Northern European ancestry. While the disease is uniquely associated with the human leukocyte antigen (HLA) –A29 phenotype and autoimmune mechanisms are thought to play an important role in its pathogenesis, its etiology remains unknown. Indeed, important questions remain in our understanding of BSRC with respect to its pathogenesis, epidemiology, optimal treatment regimens, prognosis, including predictors of remission and relapse, and in monitoring of disease progression and response to therapy with electroretinographic and psychophysical testing as well as established and emerging imaging modalities.

Pathogenesis

BSRC is unique in having the strongest association between an HLA and human disease reported to date, with up to 96% of patients being HLA-A29 positive suggesting the central importance of this molecule for disease susceptibility.[1] However, the inciting antigen is unknown and the exact role of HLA-A29 in the pathogenesis of the disease is not well understood. Indeed, there is paucity information as to the specific factors which initiate and drive ocular inflammation in humans. It has been suggested that an autoinflammatory response results from presumed molecular mimicry initiated either by prior microbial infection or other damaging factors and that HLA-A29 cross-reactive proliferative responses directed against retinal antigens could lead to loss of immunological tolerance and development of autoimmunity in BSRC.[2]

An infectious etiology has been proposed in the pathogenesis of BSRC given clustering of the disease in certain regions of Holland, Belgium, and France, either by initiating an immune response directly to the microbe itself or through molecular mimicry in a genetically predisposed individual, facilitating the presentation of autoantigen to T cells by the HLA-A29 molecule. While antibodies to *Borrelia burgdorferi* were found in 4 of 11 HLA-A29 positive patients with BSRC in one study, there is no conclusive evidence for a direct role for Lyme disease pathogenesis of this disease.[3]

The spontaneous development of a retinopathy resembling BSRC in HLA-A29 transgenic mice after 6 months of age suggests that the molecule itself plays a role in disease pathogenesis. In this model, the level of cell surface expression of HLA-A29, as well as the presence or absence of human beta 2-microglobulin, did not influence the frequency of retinopathy, suggesting that HLA-A29 itself does not mediate risk by presenting antigen to the immune system. As BSRC is a disease of older individuals in humans, it is of interest that younger transgenic mice did not develop disease, raising important questions as to role of ageing in the pathogenesis of inflammation in this disease.

While not specific to BSRC, in vitro immune responsiveness to retinal soluble antigen (S-Ag), now known as arrestin-1, and to interphotoreceptor retinoid binding protein (IRBP) have been demonstrated in a high percentage of BSRC patients.[4,5] Two peptides derived from the carboxyl-terminal sequences of human retinal soluble antigen (S-Ag) bind efficiently to HLA-A29 which may help in prediction of T-cell epitopes from retinal autoantigens implicated in BSRC.[6] Additionally, the histopathologic findings of one eye from a BSRC patient with immune responsiveness to retinal S-Ag were similar to those found in monkeys with S-Ag induced uveitis [7] while those from another HLA-A-29 patient were strikingly similar to those found in HLA-A29 transgenic mice.[8]

As its name implies, BSRC is a disease involving both the retina and choroid. While clinically it may be difficult to determine which level is affected primarily, histopathologic, electroretinographic, and imaging studies of patients with BSRC suggest that the inner retina and choroid may be affected differentially and in the earlier stages of the disease. The role of S-Ag and IRBP in disease pathogenesis must be reconciled with their location in the outer retina, suggesting that they may not be the primary inciting antigens; rather, the immune response to these antigens may be an epiphenomenon in which these proteins are released by inflammation or infection later in the disease and become autoantigens which propagate the autoimmune response.

The presence of HLA-A29 does not fully explain the full expression of disease, experimentally or in clinical experience. Not all transgenic mice develop disease, and in humans, the disease remains rare despite the fact that 7 % of the Caucasian population is HLA-A29 positive. While disease susceptibility appears linked to the HLA-A29 molecule, irrespective of subtype, other genetic or acquired factors not linked to the major histocompatibility complex (MHC) are also likely to be involved in disease development given the low prevalence of BSRC in the HLA-A29 positive population.

Recently, specific allelic combinations of the killer cell immunoglobulin-like receptor (KIR) gene, which encode for inhibitory and activating receptors expressed on human natural killer (NK) cells and some T cells, including CD8 + T lymphocytes, which are important in both innate and adaptive immunity, have been shown to confer significant risk for the development disease in HLA-A29 positive patients with BSRC while other compound genotypes were relatively protective. [9] These genes may contribute to the pathogenesis of BSRC by activating NK cells and T-cell subsets against intraocular self-antigens.

The preponderance of experimental and clinical evidence supports the notion of BSRC as a T-cell mediated autoimmune disease associated with HLA-A29; cyclosporine A (CSA), a specific inhibitor of CD4+ T cell function, has been shown to be effective in both the inhibition of S-Ag induced experimental autoimmune uveitis (EAU)[7] and in the treatment of BSRC patients.[10] Most recently, T helper 17 (TH 17) cells, a subset of CD4+ lymphocytes which secrete mainly interleukin 17 (IL-17) and play an important role in a variety of autoimmune diseases, including rheumatoid arthritis[11] and Crohn disease[12], have been implicated in the pathogenesis of BSRC. In a cohort study of 95 patients with BSRC and 25 normal controls, 41 % had significantly elevated serum levels of IFN-γ, but not IL-17 or IL 23 using a standard ELISA of 3 cytokines, suggesting a predominant role of Th1 over Th17 cell-mediated responses in the pathogenesis of this disease.[13]

In contrast, a multiplex immunoassay for the detection of 23 immune mediators in paired aqueous humor (AqH) and serum samples of 16 patients with BSRC and 11 age related cataract controls, the levels of IL-17, IL-2, IL-1β, IL-6 and TNF-α were elevated in the intraocular fluid but not in the serum, with significant positive correlation between IL-17 and both IL-2 and IL-23 and between IL-2 and IL-23.[14] The presence of elevated intraocular proinflammatory and T-cell associated cytokines suggests the novel pathogenic concept that an organ specific, Th17, cell-mediated process may be important in the pathogenesis of BSRC.

Similarly, a recent study provides complimentary information on peripheral levels of 20 immune mediators in the serum of 17 BSRC patients measured during different phases of disease activity and therapy employing quantitative, multiplex immunoassay with 12 healthy volunteers serving as controls.[15] Newly diagnosed BSRC patients with active disease, naïve to systemic immunomodulatory therapy (IMT) (n=4) exhibited significantly elevated and positively correlated serum levels of IL-21, IL-23 and TGF-β1, three of the four key cytokines which are known to be necessary for Th17 differentiation. While the fourth cytokine, IL-6, was not elevated, alternative pathways exist where either IL-21 or IL-23 together with TGF-β1 may promote Th-17 differentiation independent of IL-6.[16-18] In contrast, among BSRC patients who were on systemic IMT or who were in remission (n=13), there was no significant difference in the serum levels of immune mediators as compared to controls. While IL-23 was not found to be elevated in the AqH of BSRC patients in the previously cited study, neither IL-21 nor TGF-β1 were included in the multiplex assay.[14]

Finally the role of regulatory T cells (Tregs), which are important in the development of certain systemic autoimmune disorders such as rheumatoid arthritis[19] and systemic lupus erythematosus[20] and in selected ocular diseases including Behcet's disease[21] and Vogt-Koyanagi-Harada-syndrome[22], may be relevant in the maintenance of or escape from ocular self-tolerance in patients with BSRC. A pilot case control study of 5 patients with active treatment naïve BSRC, showed that the percentage of CD4+ CD25+Foxp3+ Tregs was significantly lower than in controls, whereas there was no difference between CD4+ CD25+ Tregs in both groups.[23]

Taken together, these studies support the notion that peripheral cytokines (IL-21, IL-23 and TGF-β1) necessary for Th17 cell differentiation may promote, amplify and maintain a chronic, intraocular Th17 cell-mediated autoimmune response in patients with active BSRC. The mechanism of which chorioretinal-specific targeting of Th17 cell-mediated inflammation occurs in BSRC remains to be elucidated, raising many more questions for further study. Is it not surprising that inflammation restricted to the eye would be associated with elevated cytokines in the peripheral blood? Are there genetic variations in the receptors for IL-21, IL-23, or TGF-β1 in patients with BSRC and is there a defective negative feedback loop in the modulation of Th17 cell activity? Is it possible that both Th1 and Th17 cell-mediated mechanisms are operative in BSRC as has been proposed in other autoimmune diseases and what is the nature of this interaction? [22] How do Tregs modulate these immunologic pathways?

In terms of clinical management, these findings underscore the importance of systemic therapy in BSRC, suggesting not only new strategies for targeted treatment, but also new insight into the determinants of and markers for the induction of sustained remission. Will elevated levels of these cytokines predict recalcitrant disease or presage inflammatory relapse? Will targeting one or more of these cytokines at various points of the Th17 cell-mediated pathway with specific biologic antagonists be more efficacious than standard IMT in the more immediate management of intraocular inflammation associated with BSRC? More important, can the active phenotype of Th17 cells and the production of proinflammatory cytokines (IL-17) be modulated in such a way to reestablish immunologic tolerance and achieve sustained remission independent of chronic therapy? Dysfunction of Tregs as measured by flow cytometry may likewise be valuable in predicting inflammatory recurrence, monitoring disease progression and response to therapy and offer new targets for targeted treatment strategies both in the short term and in an effort to achieve drug-free remission.

Epidemiology

A peculiar aspect of the epidemiology of BSRC is its essential restriction to the Caucasian population. Sequencing of the Class I region has revealed more than 20 HLA-A29 subtypes, the most common being HLA-A29.2, and HLA-A29.1, the frequency and distribution of each varying with ethnicity.[24] Among HLA-A29 positive healthy white patients of Northern European extraction, the HLA-A29.2 subtype is present in approximately 80-100%, whereas the HLA-A29.1 subtype is found more commonly among populations from Southeast Asia where BSRC is absent or extremely rare.[25] While case reports exist among Hispanic[26] and African American patients in the USA,[27] and from Japan[28], the disease is virtually nonexistent in Asia and the Indian subcontinent. The differential distribution of HLA-A29.2 and HLA-A29.1 among whites and Asians respectively has been cited as an explanation for the selective development of BSRC in patients for Northern European descent, with HLA-A29.2 thought to confer significant risk for the development of disease, while a "resistance motif" has been invoked in association with HLA-A29.1.[29,30] In the United States, the gene frequency of HLA-29.2 is 4.34% in whites, 3.57% in African Americans, and 4.91% in Hispanics and 0.42% in Asian Americans.[31] Corresponding gene frequencies for HLA-A29.1 include 0.19% in whites, 0.21% in Hispanics and 0.125% in Asian Americans. The low frequency of HLA-A29.2 in Asian Americans may partially explain the paucity of reported cases in this group; however, it does not among African Americans and Hispanics who appear strikingly protected from the disease. Recently, high resolution DNA typing of HLA-A29 among 20 patients with BSRC failed to support a protective role for HLA-A29.1 as both HLA-A29.1 and HLA-A29.2 were associated with disease.[32] Likewise, HLA-A29.1 has been reported in 2 white patients with a clinical diagnosis of BSRC; the HLA-A29.1 haplotype for white patients and Asian healthy subjects being identical, together with HLA-A29.1 and HLA-A29.2 complotypes. In addition, susceptibility to BSRC seemed to be located in the microsatellites near the locus HLA-A, and not on the HLA-A29 molecule itself.[24,33] These data suggest that heretofore unidentified factors, not linked to the HLA allele, are either protective in Asians, Hispanics and Africans or conversely, trigger autoimmune reactivity in whites.

Diagnosis

The presence of HLA-A29 is not an absolute criterion for the diagnosis of BSRC.[34] While up to 96 % of patients in the reported literature are HLA-A29 positive, based largely on antibody-based HLA typing, the positive predictive value of this test is less than 50% given low prevalence of BSRC among patients with posterior uveitis (7%) and so, routine screening is discouraged as the diagnosis of BSRC would be more often incorrect based on this test alone.[35] On the other hand, for patients with bilateral multifocal choroiditis and clinical features consistent with a diagnosis of BSRC, the negative predictive value of HLA-29 typing (99%) may be useful as it may suggest alternative diagnoses such as sarcoidosis or choroidal lymphoma in the correct clinical context. While false negative antibody-based HLA-A29 typing has been reported in 2 patients with BSRC[36], the more widespread availability of polymerase chain reaction (PCR) based techniques should eliminate these outliers. The question remains, do bona fide cases of HLA-A29 negative BSRC exist, and if so, are there important differences with respect to their prognosis and management as compared to those who HLA-A29 positive? While their number of these patients is bound to be exceedingly small making this question difficult to study, differential expression of peripheral and intraocular cytokine levels and Tregs profiles may shed light on this issue.

Treatment

When to initiate therapy, the optimal therapeutic regimen, and the duration of such treatment are important issues in the management of BSRC. While it has been suggested that as many as 20% of patients with birdshot may have self-limited disease[26], long-term follow-up suggests a course marked by multiple inflammatory exacerbations and progressive visual loss replete with structural complications and global retinal dysfunction over the long-term independent previous oral corticosteroid therapy.[37-40] Given this guarded visual prognosis and uncertain natural history, the early introduction of steroid sparing immunomodulatory therapy (IMT) has been advocated in the treatment of BSRC as extended treatment is anticipated in most patients.[41] Indeed, numerous studies have demonstrated that both preservation of visual function with a reduction of inflammation, macular edema, and preservation of global retinal integrity as well as the induction of long-term remission is possible patients with BSRC managed in this fashion.[10,26,39,40,42-44]

Certainly highly symptomatic patients with BSRC, especially those who present with or develop vitritis, retinal vasculitis, macular edema, or evidence of peripheral retinal dysfunction should be treated as described above. The situation is not as clear in the minimally symptomatic individual who presents with a classical funduscopic appearance of BSRC, no clinically apparent inflammation, absent structural complications, full visual field (VF), normal electroretinogram (ERG) and excellent visual acuity. It may be difficult to convince and/or inappropriately commit such a patient to an extended course of IMT at this point in their disease; such therapy is not entirely benign. Imaging modalities such as fluorescein angiography (FA) and indocyanine green angiography (ICGA) are very sensitive in detecting subclinical chorioretinal inflammation which may influence one's decision to treat and the institution of IMT has been shown to stabilize and even reverse both VF and ERG abnormalities associated with BSRC, which may occur even in the absence of clinically overt signs of inflammation. The question remains as to when should IMT be optimally commenced to provide the greatest long-term visual benefit while minimizing the risk for the individual patient. Prospective data are needed with respect to the rate of progression to reversible structural damage in BSRC which may provide some guidance as to exactly when to commence IMT in an effort to arrest the progression of disease before the development of irreversible visual impairment.

There is no consensus as to the optimal treatment regimen or duration of therapy for patients with BSRC. Corticosteroids are typically employed in the management of the more acute inflammatory manifestations of the disease and may be administered systemically, as bridging therapy until systemic IMT becomes effective, or as periocular and/or intravitreal injections for the treatment of acute or recurrent macular edema. Systemic corticosteroids are of inconsistent efficacy over the long run when used as chronic monotherapy requiring unacceptably high maintenance doses with the not infrequent development of serious steroid -associated adverse effects.

Systemic IMT options include anti-metabolites, T-cell transduction/calcineurin inhibitors, intravenous immunoglobulin (IVIg) and the emerging use of other biologic therapies alone or in combination.

In an initial retrospective study of 19 patients with BSRC and in the subsequent study of 28 in patients from the same institution treated with very low initial doses of cyclosporine (2.5 mg/kg/day) alone or in combination with antimetabolites (methotrexate, azathioprine, mycophenolate mofetil) or daclizumab, a favorable visual outcome, inflammatory control, stabilization of ERG parameters, and the absence of demonstrable nephrotoxic side effects were achieved.[10,43]

Similarly, a recent retrospective analysis of 76 HLA-A29 patients with BSRC, 46 of whom were followed for 5 years and 18 for more than 10 years, demonstrated that visual outcomes were better for those treated with methotrexate (MTX) as compared to untreated individuals and cortico-steroid-based regiments.[45]

While the use of MTX or cyclosporine alone may be superior to the long-term use of systemic corticosteroids in the treatment of BSRC, monotherapy with cyclosporine, in our experience, has been associated with need for exceedingly prolonged therapy with the recurrences of inflammation with tapering of this medication.

In an effort to achieve durable remission of inflammation, the combination of cyclosporine or mycophenolate mofetil (MM) has been exploited in 49 patients (98 eyes), over a mean follow up time of 65 months. At the 1-year time point, vitreous inflammatory scores, the presence of angiographic leakage, but not the presence of cystoid macular edema (CME), were significantly reduced from baseline with 67 % (31/46) patients achieving inflammatory control with no deterioration of ERG indices. All of these patients were able to maintain inflammatory remission off any kind of corticosteroids after the 1 year follow-up.[46]

For patients with inflammation refractory to conventional IMT, biological agents such as IVIG [47] and daclizumab[48,49] had been successfully employed in a small series of patients, although the latter agent is no longer available. The use of monoclonal antibodies to tumor necrosis factor (TNF-α) is an emerging treatment alternative to conventional IMT, either alone or in combination. In a recent retrospective study of 22 patients with BSRC refractory to conventional IMT treated with infliximab, inflammatory control was achieved in 81.8% and 88.9% of patients at six months and the one year follow-up respectively. Similarly, the rate of CME decreased from 22.7% at baseline to 13.9% at 6 months and to 6.7% at 12 months while the percentage of patients with a VA $\geq$ 20/40 increased from 84.1% at baseline to 91.7% and 94.4% at the six months and one year respectively.[50] Over the course of the study, 3 patients had active inflammation during therapy and 6 patients discontinued infliximab due to adverse effects.

The sustained release fluocinolone acetonide (FA) implant (Retisert®) may be a viable alternative for patients with BSRC who are unable to tolerate systemic corticosteroids or IMT.[51-53] While highly effective in the control of inflammation, reduction of CME, stabilization and /or improvement of vision and reducing the need for systemic IMT, the decision to employ this modality as initial therapy should be tempered by the universal development of cataract and a more robust intraocular pressure response to the FA implant in eyes with BSRC than in those with other types of posterior and panuveitis. Specifically, there was a statistically significant increase in intraocular pressure during the first 4 months following FA implantation as well as a higher percentage of eyes requiring glaucoma surgery and after a shorter time period following FA implantation (0.42/eye-year vs. 0.11/eye-year; median time to glaucoma surgery: 15.5 months vs. 31.5 months respectively, hazard ratio, 3.4; 95% confidence interval, 1.0-10.8, P = 0.04).[53]

While there is consensus that the early introduction of steroid-sparing IMT offers the best strategy for the long-term control of inflammation and preservation of visual function, the choice drug and the regimen employed must be individualized to the patient with consideration given to both their medical status as well as to the availability and cost of these medications. An antimetabolite is generally commenced together with systemic corticosteroids to treat the more acute manifestations of the disease; however, which antimetabolite is superior as initial therapy is not known. In the event of inflammatory recurrence while on an antimetabolite, cyclosporine or tacrolimus may be added as combination therapy. Whether sequential or initial combined therapy of an antimetabolite and a calcineurin inhibitor is most efficacious in an effort to achieve durable remission requires further prospective study. Should the inflammation recur despite combined IMT, therapy may be advanced to the available biologic agents such IVIg or TNF inhibitors with the discontinuation of cyclosporine or tacrolimus.

The demonstration of IL-17, IL-2, IL-1β and TNF-α in the AcH of patients with BSRC supports use of infliximab and daclizumab in this disease and raises the possibility for the therapeutic potential of anti-IL-17 therapy. Likewise the presence of IL-21, IL23, and TGF-β1 in the peripheral blood of patients with active, treatment naïve BSRC suggests a therapeutic rationale for the upstream or downstream targeting one or more of the cytokines involved in the Th17 cell-mediated inflammation with available or emerging biologic antagonists such as ustekinumab.[15] Whether such targeted biologic therapy is superior to standard IMT in the management of established intraocular inflammation and whether the active phenotype of Th17 cells and the production of proinflammatory cytokines (IL-17) be modulated in such a way to reestablish immunologic tolerance and achieve sustained remission independent of chronic therapy are important avenues for investigation moving forward.

Prognosis

BSRC is a chronic progressive disease with the potential for significant visual impairment due to both structural complications (CME) and diffuse retinal dysfunction with the duration of disease being a statistically significant risk factor for both. In some eyes, central visual acuity may be preserved until late in the disease course with significant irreversible peripheral retinal damage. Reported incidence rates for the development of vision loss to 20/50 or worse and to 20/200 or worse are 13% and 4 % per eye-year (EY) respectively. [42] Likewise, CME, with central visual loss, occurs at 10% per EY. The use of long-term IMT results in an 83% reduction in CME,[42] may improve and/or stabilize VF[54,55] and ERG parameters,[43,46,56-58] and in some cases, produce long-term remission in patients with BSRC.[46]

There are no prospective data with respect to rates of relapse and remission in patients with BSRC, as well as to the optimal duration of therapy with IMT to achieve this goal. The Standardization of Uveitis Nomenclature (SUN) working group has defined the term remission as inactive disease for ≥ 3 months after discontinuation of all treatments for ocular inflammation; however, this definition is clearly limited with respect to BSRC given its protracted course and the insidious nature of the development of visual dysfunction.[41] More clinically meaningful categories for clinical remission derived from those suggested for juvenile idiopathic arthritis (JIA) may be more congruent with the overall treatment goals for patients with inflammatory ocular disease in general and those with BSRC in particular and include: clinical remission, defined as inactive disease for 6 months on medication; and durable remission, defined as inactive disease off all IMT for 1 year.[59,60] Indeed, among 399 patients with inflammatory ocular disease treated at the Massachusetts Eye Research and Surgery Institution (MERSI) with systemic IMT, 50 were in durable remission as so defined, with 30% requiring at least 2 years of therapy to achieve this goal. Twenty percent remained in remission off IMT between 2 and 5 years, while 18% were in remission for more than 5 years after the discontinuation of therapy. Included in this cohort were 4 HLA-29 positive BSRC patients treated with cyclosporine in combination with mycophenolate all of whom exhibited a mean BCVA of 20/40 and had been in remission, off all medication for between 4 and 18 years. [61]

Monitoring

The treatment endpoints, and so, the determinants of relapse and remission as well as the effective evaluation of existing and novel treatment strategies in BSRC hinge on the accurate assessment and monitoring of disease activity and severity in patients with BSRC; however, there is no consensus on how to best achieve this. Given that the typical clinical indices for inflammatory activity are clearly inadequate alone for assessment of BSRC activity, a multifaceted approach employing electroretinographic and psychophysical testing, together with multimodal imaging modalities, is currently employed and highly recommended. Refinements in and standardization of the existing protocols for both ERG and VF testing, including the optimal type of perimetry, will be of value from both a clinical and research perspective; however, there are practical questions as to how they might be best integrated into clinical practice. Likewise, questions remain as to which combinations of established and emerging imaging modalities are best suited for monitoring disease activity and as to whether a BSRC phenotype may be discerned on early imaging. Finally, as previously mentioned, peripheral cytokine levels may prove to be valuable markers in monitoring disease progression, predicting inflammatory recurrence and/or recalcitrant disease as well as the response to therapy.

Full Field Electroretinography and Psychophysical Testing

Full field electroretinography and perimetry have proven invaluable in the longitudinal follow-up of patients with BSRC for detection of global retinal dysfunction and peripheral retinal abnormalities respectively in patients with BSRC. As previously noted, the institution of IMT has been shown to stabilize and even partially reverse both VF and ERG abnormalities associated with BSRC which may occur even in the absence of clinically overt signs of inflammation.[43,46,54-58]

Prolongation of the 30 Hz flicker implicit time on the full field ERG testing has emerged as the single most important proxy marker for monitoring disease patients with BSRC as it has been consistently correlated with disease activity, visual acuity, and may improve or stabilize with treatment while predicting relapse with tapering of IMT.[56-58] Likewise, perturbations in other ERG parameters such as the dim rod scotopic b wave and bright scotopic b wave amplitudes correlate with disease severity (night blindness) and treatment failure with IMT taper respectively.[56] While retrospective data suggest that longer treatment intervals and perhaps more intensive therapy with alternative IMT may achieve better inflammatory control, prospective evaluation of the incremental changes in these ERG parameters will be of value not only in validating this impression, but also, in the management of patients between clinic visits.[62] Practically, ERG testing may present logistical problems for both clinicians and patients where such expertise is not readily available.

In contrast, VF testing as a direct measure of both central and peripheral visual function is more widely available. Abnormalities on Humphrey visual field (HVF) testing were present in 62% of 80 patients with BSRC at baseline with the most common patterns being multiple foci and arcuate defects.[63] While mean deviation scores correlated with patient symptoms (blurred vision, nyctalopia and poor contrast sensitivity), and less so with visual acuity, VF abnormalities were observed in patients with normal visual acuity, underscoring the importance of monitoring peripheral retinal function in patients with BSRC. Moreover, total deviation was correlated with disappearance of the inner segment (IS)/outer segment (OS) band on time domain OCT. Goldmann visual field (GVF) defects (I-4 isopter) were present in 75% of 24 BSRC patients within 6 months of presentation with continued VF loss among those off treatment while some degree of reversibility for those receiving IMT. [54]

The progression of VF defects over time in association with disease activity[26,37,40,64] and their improvement under systemic IMT[54,55] suggests that standardized evaluations may provide data that are useful in the longitudinal management of these patients. It has been suggested that GVF testing is more sensitive than HVF protocols in the evaluation of BSRC patients although this has not been studied in large groups of patients.[54] Certainly VF testing is fraught with inconsistency due to the inherent introduction of subjectivity on the part of the patient; however, GVF testing is additionally dependent on the expertise of the technician performing the test and is less widely available than HVF testing. Similarly, while it has been suggested that ERG testing may be more sensitive in the detection of early retinal dysfunction than VF testing, practical matters of time, cost and access to available expertise of such testing must be considered. Monitoring with each modality on an alternate basis (every 6 months) may be a reasonable compromise.

Multimodal Imaging

Multimodal imaging [fluorescein angiography (FA), indocyanine green angiography (ICGA), ocular coherence tomography (OCT), and fundus autofluorescence (FAF)] in patients with BSRC has demonstrated that the inner and outer retina, retinal pigment epithelium (RPE) and choroid are all involved, albeit differentially, in this disease and are widely employed both to monitor and to guide therapy. Questions remain as to which combinations of established and emerging imaging modalities are best suited for monitoring disease activity and as to whether there exists a BSRC phenotype based on early imaging.

Fluorescein Angiography (FA)

Fluorescein angiography yields inconsistent findings and typically fails to highlight the birdshot lesions themselves. The angiographic heterogeneity of these lesions seems to depend on their age and associated degree of activity, as well as on the presence of many lesions at different stages of evolution within the same eye. More important, FA may reveal critical components of active disease including retinal vasculitis, subtle macular edema, optic nerve head leakage, and diffuse posterior pole hyperfluorescence.[65] Late structural complications of BSRC include retinal vascular attenuation, optic atrophy, epiretinal membrane formation[66,67] and the uncommon occurrence of choroidal neovascularization, the latter best visualized by FA.[68,69] The arteriovenous transit time is frequently prolonged in BSRC and it has been suggested that this finding may have diagnostic value in comparison to other posterior uveitic entities. Employing concurrent FA and ICGA, this finding has been reinterpreted in the light of the nearly normal transit time seen on ICGA versus the prolonged transit time measured on FA, attributable to extreme leakage of fluorescein dye from retinal arterioles and diffusion into the surrounding tissue prior to entering the venous circulation and to the more protein-bound, and hence, intravascular ICG. [65,70] For this reason, a timed transit should be performed in patients with BSRC. The overriding utility of both standard and wide-field FA may be in the detection of clinically unapparent retinal vascular leakage, providing a highly sensitive index for active inflammation and may even reveal a BSRC phenotype in the early stages of the disease. Indeed, retinal vascular leakage as demonstrated by FA may be associated with decreased visual acuity (VA) in eyes with a normal OCT.[71]

Indocyanine green angiography (ICGA)

Indocyanine green angiography discloses multiple hypofluorescent spots in the mid phase of the study, distributed around choroidal vessels, which may correspond to funduscopic lesions but are typically more numerous than those appreciated on clinical examination or on FA. Some areas of patchy hyperfluorescence observed on FA were not seen to correspond to the hypofluorescent dots on ICGA suggesting that the retina and choroid are differentially affected in this disease.[72] Indocyanine green angiography may be valuable diagnostically in patients with lightly pigmented fundi and very early in the course of the disease where hypofluorescent dots are readily visualized by ICGA but the lesions themselves are not apparent clinically, on color photography or on FA.[65] Patients with recent active disease may also have fuzzy, indistinct choroidal vessels and late-diffuse choroidal hyperfluorescence.[65] Both of these findings as well as the hypofluorescent dots not corresponding to window defects on FA have been reported to respond to therapy to some degree.[65,72] While providing insight into the choroidal inflammatory component of this disease, the precise use of ICGA in monitoring patients with BSRC awaits prospective study.

Fundus autofluorescence (FAF)

Fundus autofluorescence (FAF) imaging is a relatively new, non-invasive, in-vivo modality that exploits the autofluorescence properties associated with lipofuscin accumulation within RPE cells and that of other fluorophores within the outer retina and subretinal space. It provides complimentary information with respect RPE structure and function that may not be apparent with other imaging modalities and so, offer new insights into disease pathogenesis for monitoring progression.[73] FAF findings in BSRC include discrete areas of hypoautofluorescence (hypoAF) due to RPE atrophy; however there appears to be a non-uniform correspondence between these spots and the birdshot lesions seen biomicroscopically.[74,75] RPE atrophy, as visualized by FAF, is seen both in areas of hypopigmented lesions and in areas where there are no such lesions suggesting that choroid and RPE (outer retina) may be differentially and independently affected. Likewise, the presence of linear hypoAF streaks, corresponding to visible changes at the level of the RPE along retinal blood vessels in some patients, reinforces the notion that retinal vascular inflammation plays an independent role in mediating inflammatory damage to the RPE. Finally, areas of placoid macular hypoautofluorescence indicative of RPE atrophy have been significantly correlated with visual acuity of 20/50 or worse and with decreased mean foveal thickness.[74] With respect to disease monitoring, it will be of interest to learn whether these FAF findings are dynamic; changing with the progression of disease or modifiable with treatment.

Ocular Coherence Tomography (OCT)

Ocular coherence tomography is an invaluable noninvasive tool in the detection, quantification and longitudinal management of cystic, intraretinal and subretinal fluid associated inflammatory macular edema and choroidal neovascularization (CNV) and in the delineation of other structural abnormalities including, epiretinal membranes (ERM) and vitreomacular traction (VMT), in patients with BSRC.[76] At baseline, 31% of 122 eyes with BSRC were found to have macular edema using time-domain OCT.[71]

High resolution, spectral domain OCT (SD-OCT) provides more precise anatomic detail of both inner and outer retinal anatomy including the clear identification of the external limiting membrane (ELM), the photoreceptor IS/OS junction, and the RPE/Bruch's membrane complex, the integrity of each being potentially predictive of reversible and irreversible macular changes; however, there are few studies detailing these finding in patients with BSRC. Macular thinning and disruption of the photoreceptor IS/OS junction has been noted using both time domain and spectral domain OCT and had been associated with decreased visual acuity (VA), contrast sensitivity and portends a poor visual prognosis.[71,77,78] Indeed, among 14 eyes of 7 patients with longstanding BSRC, macular atrophy as measured by SD-OCT was correlated with poor VA and depressed mfERG foveal responses.[78] Macular thinning was associated with a loss of thickness of the segment subtending the proximal border of the outer plexiform layer and the Bruch-membrane-choroid interface suggesting that macular atrophy in BSRC occurs largely in the outer retina.[78,79] The mfERG was abnormal even among those patients without evidence of macular atrophy on SD-OCT suggesting that mfERG changes precede thinning on OCT damage and may serve as a sensitive surrogate marker for disease activity before the development of irreversible structural damage. Restoration of macular outer retinal architecture as visualized by SD-OCT has been described in a patient with BSRC with the institution of systemic IMT.[80]

The recent formulation of "enhanced depth imaging" (EDI) protocols[81] and extramacular image acquisition[82] with currently available SD-OCT provides high resolution visualization of the choroidal anatomy and the delineation of potentially significant structural changes outside the macula/vascular arcades respectively, heretofore unobtainable by conventional OCT. These protocols may be ideally suited for the study of uncommon chorioretinal diseases such as BSRC in which there is diffuse and differential inflammation of retina, RPE, and choroid which may not be confined entirely to the macula.

Retinal and choroidal morphology among 12 patients (24 eyes) with HLA-A29 positive BSRC was recently evaluated prospectively using a standard protocol for EDI and extramacular SD-OCT imaging and compared to that of 9 (18 eyes) normal controls.[83] Extramacular image sets revealed a spectrum of outer retinal substructure derangement ranging from focal disruption to generalized loss of the photoreceptor IS/OS junction as well as visualization of a "transition zone" in which structural abnormalities were initially seen. With generalized thinning and loss of retinal architecture, small hyper-reflective foci, thought to represent either clumping of the photoreceptors or pigment migration in response to injury, were observed in the absence of the photoreceptor IS/OS junction. Choroidal abnormalities included thinning/absence of Sattler layer, generalized atrophy, significantly reduced foveal choroidal thickness measurements relative to normal, focal choroidal hypopigmentation (increased sclera reflectivity corresponding to birdshot lesions), discrete hyper-reflective foci (proximate to birdshot lesions and thought to represent either pigment or clusters of inflammatory cells) and the presence of suprachoroidal hyporeflective space (fluid, possibly indicative of ongoing choroidal inflammation). Preliminary data from a retrospective study of 14 HLA-A29 positive BSRC patients evaluated clinically and with EDI SD-OCT indicates that both the presence and thickness of this suprachoroidal fluid band is positively correlated not only with the subjective complaint of photopsias, but also with overt signs of active inflammation , specifically, retinal vasculitis and vitritis. [84]

The use of EDI and extramacular OCT may allow improved phenotyping of posterior uveitic entities in general and BSRC in particular. Specifically, both qualitative and quantitative assessment of the IS/OS junction thickness and intensity in peripheral locations may prove valuable both in clinical practice, as a marker for disease activity and response to therapy even in situations when it appears grossly intact, and as a surrogate endpoint in clinical trials. Likewise, abnormalities in choroidal morphology, such as the presence and thickness of suprachoroidal fluid, may serve as sensitive markers for disease activity which correlates not only overt signs of inflammation (vasculitis and vitritis) but also subjective complaints (photopsias) which may influence treatment decisions. The utility of EDI in monitoring disease activity will require prospective study to determine whether and to what degree these abnormalities in choroidal morphology are modifiable with therapy. Assessment of the choroid for evidence of focal depigmentation with accompanying hyper-reflective foci may be of value diagnostically. Finally, detailed prospective evaluation of relationship between extramacular and choroidal structural abnormalities, as well as those seen on other imaging modalities, such as FAF, the presence of inflammatory activity as manifested by FA and ICGA, and their functional correlates on electroretinographic and psychophysical testing will be fruitful avenues for future investigation.

Conclusion

In summary, BSRC is a chronic, progressive sight-threatening disease, which requires the early introduction of IMT in an effort to limit ocular structural damage, preserve global visual function, and induce long-term remission. Important questions remain in our understanding of this disease with respect to its pathogenesis, epidemiology, optimal treatment, prognosis, including predictors of remission and relapse, and in monitoring of disease progression and response to therapy. Markers of active and progressive disease, which may influence treatment decisions, include not only clinical indices of intraocular inflammation, but also those seen on established and emerging imaging modalities, including FA, ICGA, OCT (with EDI) and FAF, perimetry and electroretinography. Refinements in and standardization of the existing protocols for both ERG and VF testing, including the optimal type of perimetry, will be of value from both a clinical and research perspective. Likewise, questions remain as to which combinations of established and emerging imaging modalities are best suited for monitoring disease activity and as to whether a BSRC phenotype may be discerned on early imaging. Finally, cytokine levels may prove to be valuable markers in monitoring disease progression, predicting inflammatory recurrence and/or recalcitrant disease as well as the response to therapy.

References

1. Shah KH, Levinson RD, Yu F, et al. Birdshot retinochoroidopathy. *Surv Ophthalmol.* Nov-Dec 2005;50(6):519-541.
2. Holak HM, Szymaniec S, Holak SA. The pathogenesis of birdshot retinochoroidopathy. *Surv Ophthalmol.* Jul-Aug 2006;51(4):446-447; author reply 447.
3. Suttorp-Schulten MS, Luyendijk L, van Dam AP, et al. Birdshot retinochoroidopathy and Lyme borreliosis. *Am J Ophthalmol.* Feb 15 1993;115(2):149-153.
4. Nussenblatt RB, Mittal KK, Ryan S, Green WR, Maumenee AE. Birdshot retinochoroidopathy associated with HLA-A29 antigen and immune responsiveness to retinal S-antigen. *Am J Ophthalmol.* Aug 1982;94(2):147-158.
5. de Smet MD, Yamamoto JH, Mochizuki M, et al. Cellular immune responses of patients with uveitis to retinal antigens and their fragments. *Am J Ophthalmol.* Aug 15 1990;110(2):135-142.
6. Boisgerault F, Khalil I, Tieng V, et al. Definition of the HLA-A29 peptide ligand motif allows prediction of potential T-cell epitopes from the retinal soluble antigen, a candidate autoantigen in birdshot retinopathy. *Proc Natl Acad Sci U S A.* Apr 16 1996;93(8):3466-3470.
7. Nussenblatt RB, Kuwabara T, de Monasterio FM, Wacker WB. S-antigen uveitis in primates. A new model for human disease. *Arch Ophthalmol.* Jun 1981;99(6):1090-1092.
8. Gaudio PA, Kaye DB, Crawford JB. Histopathology of birdshot retinochoroidopathy. *Br J Ophthalmol.* Dec 2002;86(12):1439-1441.

9. Levinson RD. Killer immunoglobulin-like receptor genes in uveitis. *Ocul Immunol Inflamm.* Jun 2011;19(3):192-201.
10. Vitale AT, Rodriguez A, Foster CS. Low-dose cyclosporine therapy in the treatment of birdshot retinochoroidopathy. *Ophthalmology.* May 1994;101(5):822-831.
11. McInnes IB, Schett G. Cytokines in the pathogenesis of rheumatoid arthritis. *Nat Rev Immunol.* Jun 2007;7(6):429-442.
12. Miossec P, Korn T, Kuchroo VK. Interleukin-17 and type 17 helper T cells. *N Engl J Med.* Aug 27 2009;361(9):888-898.
13. Monnet D, Batteux F, Goulvestre C, Daudin J-B, Weill B, Brezin AP. Assessment of Th17 Cells in the Pathophysiology of Birdshot Retinochoroidopathy. *Invest. Ophthalmol. Vis. Sci.* April 11, 2010 2010;51(5):3768.
14. Kuiper JJ, Mutis T, de Jager W, de Groot-Mijnes JD, Rothova A. Intraocular interleukin-17 and proinflammatory cytokines in HLA-A29-associated birdshot retinochoroidopathy. *Am J Ophthalmol.* Aug 2011;152(2):177-182 e171.
15. Yang P, Foster CS. Interleukin 21, Interleukin 23, and Transforming Growth Factor beta1 in HLA-A29-Associated Birdshot Retinochoroidopathy. *Am J Ophthalmol.* Apr 23 2013.
16. Zhou L, Ivanov, II, Spolski R, et al. IL-6 programs T(H)-17 cell differentiation by promoting sequential engagement of the IL-21 and IL-23 pathways. *Nat Immunol.* Sep 2007;8(9):967-974.
17. Korn T, Bettelli E, Gao W, et al. IL-21 initiates an alternative pathway to induce proinflammatory T(H)17 cells. *Nature.* Jul 26 2007;448(7152):484-487.

18. Manel N, Unutmaz D, Littman DR. The differentiation of human T(H)-17 cells requires transforming growth factor-beta and induction of the nuclear receptor RORgammat. *Nat Immunol.* Jun 2008;9(6):641-649.
19. Raghavan S, Cao D, Widhe M, et al. FOXP3 expression in blood, synovial fluid and synovial tissue during inflammatory arthritis and intra-articular corticosteroid treatment. *Ann Rheum Dis.* Dec 2009;68(12):1908-1915.
20. Crispin JC, Kyttaris VC, Terhorst C, Tsokos GC. T cells as therapeutic targets in SLE. *Nat Rev Rheumatol.* Jun 2010;6(6):317-325.
21. Nanke Y, Kotake S, Goto M, Ujihara H, Matsubara M, Kamatani N. Decreased percentages of regulatory T cells in peripheral blood of patients with Behcet's disease before ocular attack: a possible predictive marker of ocular attack. *Mod Rheumatol.* 2008;18(4):354-358.
22. Chen L, Yang P, Zhou H, et al. Diminished frequency and function of CD4+CD25high regulatory T cells associated with active uveitis in Vogt-Koyanagi-Harada syndrome. *Invest Ophthalmol Vis Sci.* Aug 2008;49(8):3475-3482.
23. Foster CS, Siddique SS, Amorese L, Mulki L, Suelves A. Regulatory T cells in blood of patients with birdshot retinochoroidopathy. *Ophthalmology.* Feb 2013;120(2):430 e431.
24. Donvito B, Monnet D, Tabary T, et al. Different HLA class IA region complotypes for HLA-A29.2 and -A29.1 antigens, identical in birdshot retinochoroidopathy patients or healthy individuals. *Invest Ophthalmol Vis Sci.* Sep 2005;46(9):3227-3232.
25. de Waal LP, Lardy NM, van der Horst AR, et al. HLA-A29 subtypes and birdshot retinochoroidopathy. *Immunogenetics.* 1992;35(1):51-53.

26. Gasch AT, Smith JA, Whitcup SM. Birdshot retinochoroidopathy. *Br J Ophthalmol.* Feb 1999;83(2):241-249.
27. Barondes MJ, Fastenberg DM, Schwartz PL, Rosen DA. Peripheral retinal neovascularization in birdshot retinochoroidopathy. *Ann Ophthalmol.* Aug 1989;21(8):306-308.
28. Saito W, Yamamoto S, Mitamura Y, Takeuchi S. [Birdshot retinochoroidopathy--a case report and a case study in Japanese patients]. *Nippon Ganka Gakkai Zasshi.* Apr 2002;106(4):229-235.
29. Tabary T, Lehoang P, Betuel H, et al. Susceptibility to birdshot retinochoroidopathy is restricted to the HLA-A29.2 subtype. *Tissue Antigens.* Oct 1990;36(4):177-179.
30. Tabary T, Prochnicka-Chalufour A, Cornillet P, Lehoang P, Betuel H, Cohen JH. [HLA-A29 sub-types and "Birdshot" choroido-retinopathy susceptibility: a possible "resistance motif" in the HLA-A29.1 molecule]. *C R Acad Sci III.* 1991;313(13):599-605.
31. Cao K, Hollenbach J, Shi X, Shi W, Chopek M, Fernandez-Vina MA. Analysis of the frequencies of HLA-A, B, and C alleles and haplotypes in the five major ethnic groups of the United States reveals high levels of diversity in these loci and contrasting distribution patterns in these populations. *Hum Immunol.* Sep 2001;62(9):1009-1030.
32. Levinson RD, Rajalingam R, Park MS, et al. Human leukocyte antigen A29 subtypes associated with birdshot retinochoroidopathy. *Am J Ophthalmol.* Oct 2004;138(4):631-634.

33. Donvito B, Monnet D, Tabary T, et al. A new HLA extended haplotype containing the A*2910 allele in birdshot retinochoroidopathy: susceptibility narrowed to the HLA molecule itself. *Invest Ophthalmol Vis Sci.* May 2010;51(5):2525-2528.
34. Levinson RD, Brezin A, Rothova A, Accorinti M, Holland GN. Research criteria for the diagnosis of birdshot retinochoroidopathy: results of an international consensus conference. *Am J Ophthalmol.* Jan 2006;141(1):185-187.
35. Zamecki KJ, Jabs DA. HLA typing in uveitis: use and misuse. *Am J Ophthalmol.* Feb 2010;149(2):189-193 e182.
36. Wender JD, Fu AD, Jumper JM, McDonald HR, Johnson RN, Cunningham ET, Jr. False negative antibody-based HLA-A29 typing in two patients with birdshot retinochoroidopathy. *Br J Ophthalmol.* Aug 2008;92(8):1153-1154.
37. Priem HA, Oosterhuis JA. Birdshot retinochoroidopathy: clinical characteristics and evolution. *Br J Ophthalmol.* Sep 1988;72(9):646-659.
38. Rothova A, Berendschot TT, Probst K, van Kooij B, Baarsma GS. Birdshot retinochoroidopathy: long-term manifestations and visual prognosis. *Ophthalmology.* May 2004;111(5):954-959.
39. Becker MD, Wertheim MS, Smith JR, Rosenbaum JT. Long-term follow-up of patients with birdshot retinochoroidopathy treated with systemic immunosuppression. *Ocul Immunol Inflamm.* Jul-Aug 2005;13(4):289-293.
40. Oh KT, Christmas NJ, Folk JC. Birdshot retinochoroidopathy: long term follow-up of a chronically progressive disease. *Am J Ophthalmol.* May 2002;133(5):622-629.

41. Jabs DA, Nussenblatt RB, Rosenbaum JT. Standardization of uveitis nomenclature for reporting clinical data. Results of the First International Workshop. *Am J Ophthalmol.* Sep 2005;140(3):509-516.
42. Thorne JE, Jabs DA, Peters GB, Hair D, Dunn JP, Kempen JH. Birdshot retinochoroidopathy: ocular complications and visual impairment. *Am J Ophthalmol.* Jul 2005;140(1):45-51.
43. Kiss S, Ahmed M, Letko E, Foster CS. Long-term follow-up of patients with birdshot retinochoroidopathy treated with corticosteroid-sparing systemic immunomodulatory therapy. *Ophthalmology.* Jun 2005;112(6):1066-1071.
44. Kempen JH, Altaweel MM, Holbrook JT, et al. Randomized comparison of systemic anti-inflammatory therapy versus fluocinolone acetonide implant for intermediate, posterior, and panuveitis: the multicenter uveitis steroid treatment trial. *Ophthalmology.* Oct 2011;118(10):1916-1926.
45. Rothova A, Norel AO, Los LI, Berendschot TT. Efficacy of Low-Dose Methotrexate Treatment in Birdshot Retinochoroidopathy. *Retina.* Mar 3 2011.
46. Cervantes-Castaneda RA, Gonzalez-Gonzalez LA, Cordero-Coma M, Yilmaz T, Foster CS. Combined therapy of cyclosporine A and mycophenolate mofetil for the treatment of birdshot retinochoroidopathy: a 12-month follow-up. *Br J Ophthalmol.* May 2013;97(5):637-643.
47. LeHoang P, Cassoux N, George F, Kullmann N, Kazatchkine MD. Intravenous immunoglobulin (IVIg) for the treatment of birdshot retinochoroidopathy. *Ocul Immunol Inflamm.* Mar 2000;8(1):49-57.

48. Sobrin L, Huang JJ, Christen W, Kafkala C, Choopong P, Foster CS. Daclizumab for treatment of birdshot retinochoroidopathy. *Arch Ophthalmol.* Feb 2008;126(2):186-191.
49. Yeh S, Wroblewski K, Buggage R, et al. High-dose humanized anti-IL-2 receptor alpha antibody (daclizumab) for the treatment of active, non-infectious uveitis. *J Autoimmun.* Sep 2008;31(2):91-97.
50. Artornsombudh P, Gevorgyan O, Payal A, Siddique SS, Foster CS. Infliximab Treatment of Patients with Birdshot Retinochoroidopathy. *Ophthalmology.* Nov 20 2012.
51. Srivastava SK, Nguyen QD, Callanan D, Goldstein DA, Albini TA. The Use Of The Fluocinolone Acetonide (Retisert) Implant In Patients With Birdshot Choroidopathy. *Invest. Ophthalmol. Vis. Sci.* April 22, 2011 2011;52(6):2751.
52. Rush RB, Davis J, Goldstein D, Tessler H, Lin P, Meghpara B. Birdshot Retinochoroidopathy and Fluocinolone Acetonide Intravitreal Sustained Release Devices: an Analysis of Efficacy and Complications. *Invest. Ophthalmol. Vis. Sci.* April 11, 2009 2009;50(5):6044.
53. Burkholder BM, Wang J, Dunn JP, Nguyen QD, Thorne JE. Postoperative Outcomes after Fluocinolone Acetonide Implant Surgery in Patients with Birdshot Chorioretinitis and Other Types of Posterior and Panuveitis. *Retina.* Mar 30 2013.
54. Thorne JE, Jabs DA, Kedhar SR, Peters GB, Dunn JP. Loss of visual field among patients with birdshot retinochoroidopathy. *Am J Ophthalmol.* Jan 2008;145(1):23-28.

55. de Courten C, Herbort CP. Potential role of computerized visual field testing for the appraisal and follow-up of birdshot retinochoroidopathy. *Arch Ophthalmol.* Oct 1998;116(10):1389-1391.
56. Sobrin L, Lam BL, Liu M, Feuer WJ, Davis JL. Electroretinographic monitoring in birdshot retinochoroidopathy. *Am J Ophthalmol.* Jul 2005;140(1):52-64.
57. Holder GE, Robson AG, Pavesio C, Graham EM. Electrophysiological characterisation and monitoring in the management of birdshot retinochoroidopathy. *Br J Ophthalmol.* Jun 2005;89(6):709-718.
58. Zacks DN, Samson CM, Loewenstein J, Foster CS. Electroretinograms as an indicator of disease activity in birdshot retinochoroidopathy. *Graefes Arch Clin Exp Ophthalmol.* Aug 2002;240(8):601-607.
59. Wallace CA, Ruperto N, Giannini E. Preliminary criteria for clinical remission for select categories of juvenile idiopathic arthritis. *J Rheumatol.* Nov 2004;31(11):2290-2294.
60. Wallace CA, Ravelli A, Huang B, Giannini EH. Preliminary validation of clinical remission criteria using the OMERACT filter for select categories of juvenile idiopathic arthritis. *J Rheumatol.* Apr 2006;33(4):789-795.
61. Cervantes-Castaneda RA, Bhat P, Fortuna E, Acevedo S, Foster CS. Induction of durable remission in ocular inflammatory diseases. *Eur J Ophthalmol.* Jan-Feb 2009;19(1):118-123.
62. Comander J, Loewenstein J, Sobrin L. Diagnostic testing and disease monitoring in birdshot retinochoroidopathy. *Semin Ophthalmol.* Jul-Sep 2011;26(4-5):329-336.

63. Gordon LK, Monnet D, Holland GN, Brezin AP, Yu F, Levinson RD. Longitudinal cohort study of patients with birdshot retinochoroidopathy. IV. Visual field results at baseline. *Am J Ophthalmol.* Dec 2007;144(6):829-837.
64. Fuerst DJ, Tessler HH, Fishman GA, Yokoyama MM, Wyhinny GJ, Vygantas CM. Birdshot retinochoroidopathy. *Arch Ophthalmol.* Feb 1984;102(2):214-219.
65. Fardeau C, Herbort CP, Kullmann N, Quentel G, LeHoang P. Indocyanine green angiography in birdshot retinochoroidopathy. *Ophthalmology.* Oct 1999;106(10):1928-1934.
66. Gass JD. Vitiliginous chorioretinitis. *Arch Ophthalmol.* Oct 1981;99(10):1778-1787.
67. Ryan SJ, Maumenee AE. Birdshot retinochoroidopathy. *Am J Ophthalmol.* Jan 1980;89(1):31-45.
68. Brucker AJ, Deglin EA, Bene C, Hoffman ME. Subretinal choroidal neovascularization in birdshot retinochoroidopathy. *Am J Ophthalmol.* Jan 15 1985;99(1):40-44.
69. Godel V, Baruch E, Lazar M. Late development of chorioretinal lesions in birdshot retinochoroidopathy. *Ann Ophthalmol.* Feb 1989;21(2):49-52.
70. Guex-Crosier Y, Herbort CP. Prolonged retinal arterio-venous circulation time by fluorescein but not by indocyanine green angiography in birdshot retinochoroidopathy. *Ocul Immunol Inflamm.* Sep 1997;5(3):203-206.
71. Monnet D, Levinson RD, Holland GN, Haddad L, Yu F, Brezin AP. Longitudinal cohort study of patients with birdshot retinochoroidopathy. III. Macular imaging at baseline. *Am J Ophthalmol.* Dec 2007;144(6):818-828.

72. Herbort CP, Probst K, Cimino L, Tran VT. Differential inflammatory involvement in retina and choroid in birdshot retinochoroidopathy. *Klin Monbl Augenheilkd.* May 2004;221(5):351-356.
73. Schmitz-Valckenberg S, Holz FG, Bird AC, Spaide RF. Fundus autofluorescence imaging: review and perspectives. *Retina.* Mar 2008;28(3):385-409.
74. Koizumi H, Pozzoni MC, Spaide RF. Fundus autofluorescence in birdshot retinochoroidopathy. *Ophthalmology.* May 2008;115(5):e15-20.
75. Giuliari G, Hinkle DM, Foster CS. The spectrum of fundus autofluorescence findings in birdshot retinochoroidopathy. *J Ophthalmol.* 2009;2009:567693.
76. Gallagher MJ, Yilmaz T, Cervantes-Castaneda RA, Foster CS. The characteristic features of optical coherence tomography in posterior uveitis. *Br J Ophthalmol.* Dec 2007;91(12):1680-1685.
77. Kappel PJ, Monnet D, Yu F, Brezin AP, Levinson RD, Holland GN. Contrast sensitivity among patients with birdshot retinochoroidopathy. *Am J Ophthalmol.* Feb 2009;147(2):351-356 e352.
78. Birch DG, Williams PD, Callanan D, Wang R, Locke KG, Hood DC. Macular atrophy in birdshot retinochoroidopathy: an optical coherence tomography and multifocal electroretinography analysis. *Retina.* Jun 2010;30(6):930-937.
79. Forooghian F, Yeh S, Faia LJ, Nussenblatt RB. Uveitic foveal atrophy: clinical features and associations. *Arch Ophthalmol.* Feb 2009;127(2):179-186.
80. Forooghian F, Gulati N, Jabs DA. Restoration of retinal architecture following systemic immunosuppression in birdshot retinochoroidopathy. *Ocul Immunol Inflamm.* Dec 2010;18(6):470-471.

81. Spaide RF. Enhanced depth imaging optical coherence tomography of retinal pigment epithelial detachment in age-related macular degeneration. *Am J Ophthalmol.* Apr 2009;147(4):644-652.
82. Kriechbaum K, Bolz M, Deak GG, Prager S, Scholda C, Schmidt-Erfurth U. High-resolution imaging of the human retina in vivo after scatter photocoagulation treatment using a semiautomated laser system. *Ophthalmology.* Mar 2010;117(3):545-551.
83. Keane PA, Allie M, Turner SJ, et al. Characterization of birdshot retinochoroidopathy using extramacular enhanced depth optical coherence tomography. *JAMA Ophthalmol.* Mar 1 2013;131(3):341-350.
84. Birnbaum A, Fawzi A, Rifkin L, Goldstein D. Correlation between Disease Activity and Choroidal Patterns by OCT-EDI in Birdshot Retinochoroidopathy. *Invest. Ophthalmol. Vis. Sci.* June 16, 2013 2013;54(6):5204.

Chapter 14

Bridging the Gaps in Knowledge

Robert B. Nussenblatt

In being asked to offer my comments concerning how to approach the gaps in knowledge concerning Birdshot Retinochoroidopathy (BSRC), it must be understood that it is offering one point of view, it is not a consensus approach. I apologize in advance if I hurt the feelings of some; it is certainly not my intention. The problem of how to move forward is faced of course by many subspecialties, particularly those studying relatively rare diseases. It is becoming clear that some general approaches tend to repeat themselves and I think they are applicable when discussing BSRC. For this exercise it seems to be reasonable to divide the discussion between phenotype and the underlying immune aspects, often shortened and called phenotype, but we know it is far more complicated than just finding a gene. This division though accepts that Ophthalmology cannot really move forward alone to fill in the gaps we deal with in BSRC. Ophthalmologists can help significantly in dealing with the phenotype, but no more.

Dr. Vitale has very nicely outlined the problems that he sees from a clinical perspective. Permit me to expound upon these and go a bit beyond.

Phenotypes of disease - better definition of the disorder

This is clearly one of the central tasks before us and is critical. The original definition of the disease by Ryan and Maumenee (1) was described by Baarsma, Priem, and Kijlstra (2) as follows: "In 1980 Ryan and Maumenee described a new clinical entity characterized by hypopigmented spots in a typical patterned distribution in association with vitritis and retinal vasculopathy leading to cystoid macular oedema and papilloedema."The definition has been altered on several occasions. Indeed we are unable to even agree upon the name of the disorder. There are well over 100 articles discussing BSRC, with the original articles describing it as "chorioretinopathy" while others describe it as "retinochoroidopathy". This is not a subtle distinction since it has significant implications in terms of possible autoimmune driven mechanisms. I must admit that I do in fact have a preference for retinochoroidopathy, because of the strong evidence of retinal autoimmune responses based on T cell anamnestic responses and the HLA 29 character, which we will come to in a moment. Practically speaking what is enough to make the diagnosis? The findings supporting the diagnosis of birdshot retinochoroidopathy were in the original Maumenee and Ryan article: white female, late 40s to 50s with an ocular examination showing a quiet anterior chamber but vitreous inflammation but no snowbanking. In addition there was retinal vascular leakage and CME. Finally there were deep circular cream-colored lesions, mostly in the posterior pole and surrounding areas. Gass described vitiligo as part of the disorder and others have associated other systemic findings.

Clearly a consensus is needed. This consensus has begun with the SUN community, members of which are at this meeting on BSRC. The Standardization of Uveitis Nomenclature working group brought together 79 uveitis experts from 18 countries. This international workshop initially met, and discussed better ways to standardize clinical observations. Smaller groups using nominal group techniques were then used to reach consensus on particularly troublesome issues. Out of this came a standardized way in which ocular inflammatory disease is recorded and this has now become the standard. Now enhanced computational approaches have begun working on disorder definitions, including BSRC. It will be important to include this group in any decision making.

Natural history of the disease

It has been suggested that 20% of BSRC patients do well long term. That is not my experience. What I think is more important is that it is a reasonably rare disease and the definitions that circulate are variable. Different reporting investigators may not be following exactly the same patient groups. Once again, a standardized method of clinical data collection becomes absolutely critical.

Testing

Additional supportive testing is critical. Simple things sometimes are overlooked and this can be very detrimental to the patient's ocular course. One example is visual fields.

We have seen patients followed for years, who maintained good central vision and then began to have difficulty reading. Visual fields showed only a central field with marked peripheral constriction. Should other tests be added and when? Gass (3) made an observation that the fluorescein angiogram did not demonstrate the cream colored lesions as well as simple fundus photography did. Others have suggested that ICG is a good way to follow this disorder.(4) Now with enhanced angiographic visualization of the retinal vascular periphery what do changes there mean for the patient's long term visual health?

Therapy

I will return to this subject later but suffice to say this is of course a very important practical question. With BSRC being relatively rare, randomized controlled trials will be a major challenge, to say the least. Randomized controlled trials are still the recognized gold standard by which a therapeutic approach can be best evaluated. Which medication would you chose and why? We simply do not have enough information at this point to make a choice. BSRC could be included in larger studies recruiting non-infectious uveitis patients in general, but we would never completely know the potential effectiveness of a medication for BSRC. Another consideration is the length of study. Six month long studies showing "activity" of a drug really will not meet the need of the BSRC patient who needs long term therapy. With no criteria for patient definition nor guidelines to treat nor criteria for how long to treat, we are relegated to hit and miss medicine.

Laboratory needs

This leads us to the next important gap in our knowledge-Laboratory needs. In many respects these evaluations will clearly impact on the clinical/phenotype part of the disease. The important message is that while this is central to much that can be done in the future, this cannot be done by ophthalmologists. The implication of my words is that while meetings like this one certainly have their importance for patients and clinicians, in my opinion this approach will not address the central question of the underlying disease mechanism.

There are major questions that still need to be answered. We reported the strong association with HLA-A29 over 20 years ago and most clinicians will use this test to confirm their clinical diagnosis. However, we do not know the true mechanistic reason for this association. There have been associations made with other molecules known to be involved with the immune process, but frankly to date these are associations with no real insight into mechanism. These observations and the following examples really speak to the simple fact that if we are serious about closing gaps we need to engage the larger clinical immunologic community and the clinician's role will need to be secondary. I would emphasize that animal work probably will not be central to these observations. Let me give a few reasons to support this notion. The first is that the evidence accruing supports the notion that ocular inflammatory disease is a systemic disease with local manifestations. Clinically we know that even ocular inflammations which are usually localized to the eye can indeed have systemic manifestations. We certainly see evidence of immune alterations in the periphery. Indeed the story is more complicated than that. In a study we published several years ago (5) we evaluated gene expression using microarray technology of patients with several different types of non-infectious intermediate and posterior uveitis, including BSRC. Using a pathway specific cDNA microarray we evaluated 50 patients with uveitis. A total of 67 inflammation and autoimmune genes were found differentially expressed in these patients. Our goal was to identify a specific gene signature for the disease entities that we studied. Several gene patterns of expression were identified. However, to our surprise we found that different gene signatures were found in the same clinical entities. Thus, as we define phenotypes assuming that the clinical similarities reflect an underlying mechanistic similarity is probably not true. The implications are very important clinically. We may not be treating the same disease though phenotypically they seem to be. The importance for clinicians is that if we begin to define such differences we would identify patients with similar underlying immune mechanisms, and we would need fewer patients for clinical trials, and this can have important implications for those whose deal with rare diseases. A second example is the question of genetics. While genetics prepare the groundwork for immune responses, it has become increasingly clear that gene variants are not as important in understanding mechanisms. Indeed, an uncomfortable truth is that most gene variants (SNPs) are not in the coding regions of genes. An area of great interest that has recently been aggressively studied has been epigenetics. We recently reported epigenetic changes in age related macular degeneration. Newer techniques evaluating RNA expression as well as other newer technologies have completely changed how immune mechanisms, particularly those seen in humans, are now evaluated. To bridge the gaps we need to more aggressively join the larger immunologic world.

Bridging the gaps

There are probably several ways that dealing with our clinical and immune needs could be met. Since we are dealing with a relatively rare disorder a consensus amongst investigators defining the disease is absolutely needed. This initial step is mentioned in comments above. Once done, then a clinical database needs to be established. This would include the collection of psychophysical data as well. This would be linked to a specimen database collected from the same patients. This is of course easier said than done. An oversight committee needs to be appointed. Their role is to oversee the collection of data initially. However, a very important role is the need for this committee to evaluate the material being collected to assure the material is relevant and accessible. There may be new clinical tests that will be important to add to the material collected. The collection of tissue will also be of vital importance. SOPs will need to be developed to assure uniform collection of data. The creators of the tissue data base need to be aware that more than DNA will be needed. GWAS evaluations are beginning to run out of steam and other areas, such as epigenetics and RNA evaluations, are becoming more commonly performed. The committee will need to set standards for those who wish to use the information collected. This can be a real challenge. In my mind, however, if we are really serious about bridging gaps we must engage colleagues in immunology. The role of most ophthalmologists will be minimal, but it is perhaps seminal to bridging the gap. The underlying mechanism(s) will be a key element to our understanding BSRC and treating it. Engagement means reaching out and convincing immunologists that BSRC and the eye are ideal for the study of organ specific immune mechanisms, of course. We can continue to try medications that are developed for other indications. We could become lucky and find new therapies by chance or we can more systemically evaluate medications based on scientific observations. There is even a larger goal that should be our greatest objective. The disease itself develops as a consequence of a loss of peripheral immune tolerance. Reinvigorating peripheral immune privilege is a goal for many putative autoimmune disorders and should be for BSRC. The only way that this can be accomplished is for Ophthalmology to relinquish its hold on this disease and enter into the larger immune sphere. Suggestions to pursue this path have not been well received in the past.

I believe that a framework along these lines would lead to significant progress. However there are obvious obstacles, in some ways related. We are not a well-organized group and for the moment are not particularly attractive to the larger clinical immunology community, except when it comes to very specific questions. The other major factor is of course financial support for such an endeavor. Private support would be needed to begin the organizational changes outlined. This is a long term investment and many who are able to support such an endeavor may grow weary if no advances are made immediately to help a loved one with this disorder. All of this is true but closing these gaps will not occur without such an investment. It has been done in other areas of medicine.

References

1. Ryan SJ, Maumenee AE. Birdshot retinochoroidopathy. Am J Ophthalmol 1980; 89:31–45.
2. Baarsma GS, Priem HA, Kijlstra A. Association of birdshot retinochoroidopathy and HLA-A29 antigen. Curr Eye Res. 1990;9 Suppl:63-8.
3. Gass J. Vitiligious chorioretinitis. Arch Ophthalmol 1981; 99: 1778–1787.
4. Herbort CP, Probst K, Cimino L, et al. Differential inflammatory involvement in retina and choroid in birdshot retinochoroidopathy. Klin Monatsbl Augenheilkd 2004; 221(5): 351–356.
5. Li Z; Maminishkis A; Mahesh SP; Yeh S; Lew J; Lim WK; Sen HN; Clarke G; Buggage R; Miller SS; Nussenblatt RB. Gene expression profiling in autoimmune noninfectious uveitis disease. J Immunol 2008; 181:5147-57.

Made in the USA
Las Vegas, NV
04 November 2026

57423057R00138